Health Communication for Health Care Professionals

Michael P. Pagano, PhD, PA-C, is an associate professor (tenured) in the Department of Communication, Fairfield University, Fairfield, Connecticut. His areas of research interest include health communication, health care organizations, health care pedagogy, pharmaceutical marketing, electronic medical records, and interpersonal and gendered communication. He teaches numerous courses and has been an invited speaker on these topics and has published widely in all of these areas. Dr. Pagano has authored five books, all of which are on health communication, and three book chapters, including "Enhancing Communication Skills Through Simulation," published in Campbell and Daley's *Simulation Scenarios for Nurse Educators: Making It Real,* second edition (Springer Publishing Company, 2013). Dr. Pagano is the invited associate editor of the *Health Behavior & Policy Review Journal* and sits on the editorial board of the *Nursing Communication Journal.* Among other honors, he was elected Fairfield University Cura Personalis Faculty Mentor of the Year 2008 to 2009 and again in 2012 to 2013. He served 3 years as a medical corpsman in the U.S. Army, including 1 year in Vietnam as a combat medic. Dr. Pagano currently serves as thesis adviser to several graduate students. He works per diem as a physician assistant in the emergency department, Stamford Hospital, Stamford, Connecticut.

Canera L. Pagano, JD, RN, is the director of risk management at Yale New Haven Health System's Bridgeport Hospital in Bridgeport, Connecticut. She was a malpractice attorney for the defense (providers) for 7 years. She has been the director of risk management for 5 years. She has given invited lectures to health professionals on a variety of risk and legal issues, including medical malpractice, medical records, adverse events, and risk management.

Health Communication for Health Care Professionals

An Applied Approach

Michael P. Pagano, PhD, PA-C

With Chapters on Risk Management
and Medical Malpractice by

Canera L. Pagano, JD, RN

SPRINGER PUBLISHING COMPANY
NEW YORK

Springer Publishing Company, LLC
11 West 42nd Street
New York, NY 10036
www.springerpub.com

Acquisitions Editor: Margaret Zuccarini
Composition: diacriTech

ISBN: 978-0-8261-2441-8
e-book ISBN: 978-0-8261-2442-5
Instructor's Manual ISBN: 978-0-8261-2439-5
PowerPoint ISBN: 978-0-8261-2455-5

Instructor's Materials: Qualified instructors may request supplements by e-mailing textbook@springerpub.com

16 17 18 19 / 5 4 3 2 1

The author and the publisher of this Work have made every effort to use sources believed to be reliable to provide information that is accurate and compatible with the standards generally accepted at the time of publication. Because medical science is continually advancing, our knowledge base continues to expand. Therefore, as new information becomes available, changes in procedures become necessary. We recommend that the reader always consult current research and specific institutional policies before performing any clinical procedure. The author and publisher shall not be liable for any special, consequential, or exemplary damages resulting, in whole or in part, from the readers' use of, or reliance on, the information contained in this book. The publisher has no responsibility for the persistence or accuracy of URLs for external or third-party Internet websites referred to in this publication and does not guarantee that any content on such websites is, or will remain, accurate or appropriate.

Library of Congress Cataloging-in-Publication Data
Names: Pagano, Michael P., author. | Pagano, Canera L., author.
Title: Health communication for health care professionals : an applied
    approach / Michael P. Pagano.
Description: New York, NY : Springer Publishing Company, LLC, [2017] | With
    chapters on risk management and medical malpractice by Canera L. Pagano
    JD, RN. | Includes bibliographical references and index.
Identifiers: LCCN 2016020114 | ISBN 9780826124418
Subjects: | MESH: Health Communication | Professional-Patient Relations |
    Communication | Health Personnel
Classification: LCC RA427.8 | NLM WA 590 | DDC 362.1—dc23 LC record available at
https://lccn.loc.gov/2016020114

Special discounts on bulk quantities of our books are available to corporations, professional associations, pharmaceutical companies, health care organizations, and other qualifying groups. If you are interested in a custom book, including chapters from more than one of our titles, we can provide that service as well.
For details, please contact:
Special Sales Department, Springer Publishing Company, LLC
11 West 42nd Street, 15th Floor, New York, NY 10036-8002
Phone: 877-687-7476 or 212-431-4370; Fax: 212-941-7842
E-mail: sales@springerpub.com

Printed in the United States of America by Gasch Printing.

This book is dedicated to our granddaughters, Caitlin Elizabeth and Scarlett Josephine, with the hope that their futures will be enhanced by more effective interpersonal health communication, collaborative decision making, reduced health risks, and a patient-centered focus on wellness.

And to Dr. Sandy Ragan, professor emeritus, the University of Oklahoma, who took a chance working with a nontraditional health care provider turned graduate student, changed her scholarly focus and taught so many of us the importance of researching, teaching, and writing about interpersonal provider–patient interactions and improving health communication outcomes.

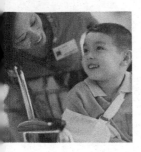

Contents

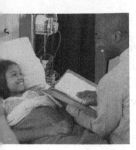

Foreword

I've been teaching both a social science–oriented health communication class and a skills-oriented communication for the health professions class for several years. I have no difficulty finding a good book for the former, but the books that are geared toward skills for health professionals tend to ignore a sophisticated conceptualization of communication processes. They tend to be based more on anecdotal evidence rather than empirical work. As I revised my plan for the course for health professionals a few years ago, I got in touch with Michael P. Pagano, as I was using his case studies book within that class and I wanted his input on the cases that coordinated most effectively with the various chapters in the other text I was using in the course. He provided very helpful feedback, and even created some individual case studies for my students and simulated patients that semester. As we communicated, he shared some ideas that I found useful for my course. This led me to say, "Why don't you write a better book for me to use as the primary text in my class?" And he did! This book is the product of that conversation and I am delighted to be able to use it in my course. Thus, I am partially responsible for this volume. I'm perfectly willing to share in the credit.

The reader will find the best of both worlds in this book. Michael, with the help of Canera L. Pagano, has a sophisticated understanding of communication processes as well as a thorough understanding of the complexities of the health care process. Most people who write in this area have only one or the other, but a good health communication book that can help health professionals requires both. Both teachers and students will benefit. The communication process and both health and health care delivery are notably intertwined. Communication is directly related to the accuracy of diagnosis and to the adequacy of information communicated by patients and care providers. Health care providers may improve provision of care by understanding and empathizing with patients more completely.

In addition, the reader of this book will find that it is replete with useful and interesting examples, reflections, discussion questions, and exercises.

This is a very interactive volume that will facilitate student engagement and learning at all levels. It focuses on both verbal and nonverbal dimensions of communication and examines the impact of all key audience characteristics on the communicative process. In each case, opportunity is provided to practice and analyze relevant skills. I am particularly pleased with the foci provided within the book on outcomes, ethics, organizational issues, malpractice, end-of-life communication, and cultural concerns. The book is simultaneously well grounded in medical knowledge and in communication theory and research. The reader will appreciate the focus on avoiding communication problems in health care.

I am delighted to be able to use this book in my class, and am proud to have been a part of talking Michael into writing it. It fills an important void in the market for professors, students, and future health care professionals. I think you will enjoy and appreciate it.

Teresa L. Thompson, PhD
Editor, *Health Communication*
Professor
University of Dayton
Dayton, Ohio

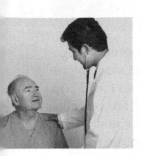

Preface

This text is intended to enhance and stimulate the exploration, effectiveness, and education of the behaviors and skills of health professions students (RN, MD, physician assistant [PA], doctor of osteopathy [DO], advanced practice registered nurse [APRN], physical therapist [PT], etc.) and practicing health care providers related to provider–patient, provider–provider, and provider–organization interpersonal, health, team, and organizational communication. According to a report from the Institute of Medicine, between 40,000 and 100,000 Americans die annually from medical errors This text is intended to highlight the fact that, at the most fundamental level, all medical errors are communication based.

Therefore, whether you want to better understand the theories that underlie the messages sent via verbal and nonverbal communication, or you want to enhance your listening, speaking, and/or interacting abilities, this book is intended to support your efforts. The primary author has more than 50 years of combined experience/expertise as a health care provider (PA, registered nurse, and army corpsman). Canera L. Pagano has more than a decade of health care/malpractice law and risk-management experience. Their diverse backgrounds cross numerous health care contexts (hospitals, clinics, surgery, OB/GYN, family practice, occupational health, emergency medicine, provider education, malpractice defense, administrative, etc.). They use these experiences to help readers apply the theories and behavioral recommendations discussed in this text to enhance providers' understanding of health communication and its role in U.S. health care delivery.

This book is intended to serve as a source of information, primarily as a stimulant for interaction, exploration, application, reflection, and self-assessment. Effective health communication is the result of a complex process that begins with understanding the theories related to various interdependent and interrelated communication disciplines (interpersonal, intercultural, small group/team, organizational, health, etc.). To assist you in better assimilating and utilizing these disciplines, each chapter provides real and/or hypothetical examples that can be assessed and analyzed. Therefore, the authors encourage you not to just read each chapter, but also to apply what you are studying to your daily interactions with patients, peers, friends, family, and so forth. The more conscious you are of how you communicate, verbally and nonverbally, in all contexts, the more likely you are to enhance your effectiveness in the most challenging and emotionally charged communication context of all—health care. Most communication between providers and patients is psychologically affected as a result of a number of predictable factors:

- Patient's fear
- Health literacy inequality
- Provider power/control (perceived and real)
- Prior experiences (patients with providers and providers with patients)

With these understandings and goals in mind, please begin your journey through this text by asking the simple question "why"? Why study health communication when you have been interacting with friends, lovers, professionals, clients, patients, and so forth for years or decades? We urge you to keep asking that very important "why" question throughout your exploration of this text and your application of the material provided. Perhaps you could seek "why" answers not to a defensive, "why do I need to study communication" query, but rather to a more reflective "why don't health care providers do more (listening, translating of medical jargon, collaborative decision making, etc.)?" Or "why do health care organizations communicate with (providers or patients or both) in such an authoritarian fashion?" The authors do their best to help you assess these difficult, but very important, questions in an effort to help you become the most effective interpersonal communicator of health care information possible.

In addition to this text, qualified instructors can obtain a Power-Point presentation and Instructor's Manual by e-mailing textbook@ springerpub.com.

Michael P. Pagano

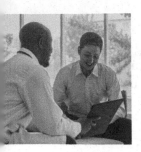

CHAPTER 1

A Brief History of U.S. Health Care

For the purpose of this text, we are going to use the following as working definitions:

- *Communication channels:* Various means for transmitting messages (verbal and/or nonverbal); includes, but is not limited to air (voice, face-to-face), mechanical/electronic (phone, Internet, etc.), written (e-mail, texts, newspapers, etc.), visual (movies, TV, etc.), and more

- *Health care provider:* Any member of the health care team who directly (or indirectly) impacts a patient's health/wellness/quality of life (e.g., doctors, nurses, advanced practice registered nurses [APRNs], physician assistants [PAs], respiratory therapists, physical therapists, and many others)

- *Intercultural communication*: How individuals communicate across cultures (e.g., American, French, Spanish, etc.), but also within and across subcultures (e.g., physicians, nurses, patients, etc.)

- *Interpersonal (also known as dyadic) communication:* Interactions between two people who know each other and share common goals (e.g., friends, lovers, family members, professionals, and a provider and a patient); not the same as an infrequent conversation between a customer and a store clerk or waitperson

- *Interpersonal relationship:* A bond between two people who share common goals that requires effective interpersonal communication to develop and/or maintain

- *Interprofessional communication:* How providers from different health care professions (MD/DO [doctor of osteopathy], RN, PA, technicians, etc.) share information, tasks, and so on

- *Intraprofessional communication:* Interactions between members of the same profession (physician–physician, RN–RN, PA–PA, physical therapist–physical therapist, etc.)

- *Organizational communication:* How institutions (e.g., hospitals, governments, health insurance payers, etc.) communicate internally with staff, providers, administrators, and externally with customers, clients, patients, vendors, and/or stake/stockholders
- *Pedagogy:* The study of teaching

HEALTH COMMUNICATION

For the purpose of this book, *health communication* is defined—using a generalist's view—as any exchange of information (verbal, nonverbal, or written) that relates to an individual's or the public's health (clinically, pedagogically, politically, professionally, institutionally, economically, commercially, legally, etc.). This broad view has been chosen to highlight the countless and complex ways health communication touches the lives of not only health care professionals and patients, but all Americans. It is important to recognize that at its core, most health communication is dyadic; however, it would be extremely shortsighted to ignore the enormous impact of organizational (especially the federal government), intercultural, and team communication on U.S. health care delivery. This book is intended to help readers understand the dynamic and complex roles health communication plays in Americans' daily lives. From wellness to illness, effective health communication is one of the keys to enhancing everyone's quality of life. And, armed with an understanding of the theories and realities of health communication for professionals, the book's goals are to encourage readers to apply their learning both in their personal and professional lives. Therefore, to begin our exploration of health communication in America—let us start at the beginning.

A HISTORICAL OVERVIEW OF HEALTH COMMUNICATION: THE FIRST AMERICAN HOSPITAL

Thanks to one of our founding fathers, organized health care in America can be traced to the first U.S. hospital. Franklin (1754) wrote *Some Account of the Pennsylvania Hospital: From Its First Rise to the Beginning.* As a cofounder of the first hospital in the 13 colonies, Franklin points out how important health care delivery was to the early settlers of Philadelphia. In addition, more than a decade later, the first American medical school was opened at the University of Pennsylvania. Therefore, health care in this country, at least from an organizational perspective, can be traced from those meager beginnings 260-plus years ago. It is important for us, in the current era of multichannel communication, to recognize the information sharing and scientific limitations that existed for the majority of American health care history. It was only within the last century that so many of the breakthroughs in science, health care, and communication all occurred. Therefore, for most of the first 150 or more years of health care in this country, providers and patients had not only rudimentary diagnostic and therapeutic options for treating illnesses and injuries, but similarly limited access to information, as well as tools for, or education about, how to best share it. Although there may have been some providers who could receive printed materials, many, if not most, learned from other providers and whatever textbooks were available. There were no phones, no electricity, and very limited postal service. In short, in this country health care education was highly restricted until after 1910 and, therefore, so too were providers' information sources. Combine the lack of clinical assessment tools and communication opportunities and it should be no surprise that the average life span in America for men and women was less than 48 years. In fact, it is a testament to our forefathers/mothers that with so little medical knowledge and health communication they were able to live as long as they did.

Reflection 1.1. With so few scientific instruments at his or her disposal, what would you hypothesize would be most important to a provider's analysis of patients' diagnostic success and why?

_____

_____

_____

_____

_____

■ IMPACT OF WARS ON HEALTH CARE DELIVERY

Although there were medical schools opening across the United States during the 18th and 19th centuries, one of the key methods for learning new diagnostic and treatment regimens during this time was to try out various procedures and tests during war time. Physicians and surgeons, starting with the American Revolution through the Spanish–American War, had no shortage of ill and injured patients and, with no real alternatives for the soldiers, they were ideally suited as research subjects. Therefore, many of the emerging methods for organizing care, triaging patients, diagnosing illnesses and injuries, and a wide variety of orthopedic and surgical procedures were conceived, practiced, and routinized in makeshift outdoor medical aid stations and surgical areas during American warfare.

■ BARTERING FOR HEALTH CARE

During America's preindustrial revolution, because of the largely agricultural society, patients and providers who were not involved in wars experienced most of their health care delivery in patients' homes. House calls, as they were known, were common and bartering was a typical way for farmers, shopkeepers, and others to pay for a doctor's services. Therefore, a bushel of potatoes might cover the cost of repairing a child's broken arm, or a small pig might be payment for delivering a baby. During this period, these methods of compensation were as primitive as much of medical education. Because many of the doctors during this time trained as apprentices by studying with a similarly trained, practicing physician, they could only learn what their mentors knew. However, prior to 1900, even in the emerging medical and nursing schools there were no real standardizations of curriculum, procedures, or policies being used or taught.

Reflection 1.2. What are three communication issues that you think contributed to the lack of standardization in health provider education from 1751 to 1900?

1. _____

2. _____

3. _____

■ A DISEASE-CENTERED APPROACH

As America evolved during the Industrial Revolution, health care too had to adapt to the changing societal landscape. With more people needed in urban areas to work in the emerging industries, the number of providers required to care for them expanded. During this same period, the federal government began to question the lack of medical standardization, licensure, and educational consistency. Based on these assessments, today's health education models were developed. The evolution of modern health care was based on a scientific model that sought to identify and treat diseases and injuries using objective assessments and data analysis. This disease-centric approach led to a standardization in medical education and licensure; the discovery of countless technological advances from the microscope, to antibiotics and x-ray machines—and throughout the 20th and into the 21st century—to vaccines, surgical robots, and gene-based therapies.

■ THE RISE AND IMPACT OF TECHNOLOGY

However, as science and technology became more normative in health care, providers became more specialized. Therefore, as x-ray machines become more common in everyday medical practice, a specialty in radiology was created to provide expert x-ray interpretation. Similarly, a specialty in pathology was perceived as critical to the burgeoning field of tissue and laboratory analyses. Over the past century, more than 120 specialties and subspecialties have developed in American health care to focus on specific anatomic and/or physiologic systems/processes. Some of these specialties include cardiology, dermatology, endocrinology, ophthalmology, urology, and so forth, all of which require post-medical school training (internship and residency) to focus on a specific anatomical (or physiological) area of study. However, there were also specialty areas developed that focused on specific disease processes: allergy, oncology, rheumatology, and so on. Although on one hand, specialization provides patients with a provider who is credentialed as an expert in a particular aspect of diagnosis, disease, and/or treatment, it also creates a number of personal and societal issues.

Reflection 1.3. Why might the term *specialist* have negative implications for patients?

_____

_____

_____

_____

_____

As will be discussed in future chapters, the expanding role and utilization of technology have impacted health care and health communication in diverse ways, for example, today there are:

- Fewer general/family practitioners graduating from medical schools
- Markedly increased health care costs
- Heightened language barriers between specialists and patients
- Frequent status disparities among providers
- Access to care inequalities

Although there is little doubt that technology and the rise in specialization and specialty care (surgical intensive care units, burn centers, coronary care units, dialysis centers, etc.) have helped increase life expectancy in America to around 76 years of age for men and 80 years of age for women, technology and specialization have also contributed to many societal problems, the most critical of which is—rising U.S. health care costs.

■ PHARMACEUTICAL CONTRIBUTIONS TO HEALTH AND COSTS

But technology is not just about developing diagnostic and treatment equipment. Another of the byproducts of the technological era is the vast advancement in pharmaceutical research and development (R&D). In the United States, beginning with the release of penicillin in the 1940s until today, the Food and Drug Administration (FDA) has approved over 1,500 prescription drugs. So in 70 years, technology has helped bring about a wide variety of treatment and/or prevention options for diverse diseases like hypertension, hypothyroidism, polio, hemophilia, osteoporosis, arthritis, and countless others. However, as with other aspects of technology, pharmaceutical advancements have come with a steep price tag. In 2013, U.S. spending on prescription drugs exceeded $325 billion. Although these products have helped expand Americans' life expectancy, the economic price has created enormous micro- and macrofiscal issues for individuals', families', and the nation's health care budget.

■ CONTEMPORARY AMERICAN HEALTH CARE AND ITS IMPACT ON HEALTH COMMUNICATION

President Obama and Congress created the 2010 Affordable Care Act in an apparent tripartite effort to reduce escalating health care costs. First, the Act was intended to get as many uninsured Americans health care coverage as possible. Second, the Act sought to reduce national health care costs through numerous steps, including the use of electronic medical/health records (EMRs) in hospitals and providers' offices. Third, the Act promoted preventive care by eliminating copays for insured citizens.

If you examine a few of the major foci of the Affordable Care Act highlighted previously, it becomes obvious the role health communication plays in America's health care delivery system. For example, without insurance, people generally have to go to a community clinic and do not see the same provider (continuity of care) from one visit to the next. This reality makes an interpersonal relationship between provider and patient less likely and thus diminishes patient trust, comfort, and, often times, adherence with recommended treatment plans. In addition, the lack of insurance and an interpersonal relationship also increases the likelihood that the next time the patient is ill she or he may go to the emergency department (ED) for care—because it is open 24/7/365 and by law cannot refuse service to anyone. But the communication exchange in an overworked ED between patient and provider is more likely to be even less interpersonal than in a busy community clinic. The Act also tried to improve access to patients' medical records for a number of communication reasons (legibility, information sharing, less duplication/redundancy, content consistency, etc.), but also for finance-related issues. Insurers (like Medicare and Medicaid, as well as private plans) wanted to be certain what services were provided and whether they met local/regional/national providers' standard of care. Therefore, health professionals' communication in an EMR becomes even more important (personally, organizationally, and for the patient) from both clinical and financial perspectives. Finally, because even with insurance many patients cannot afford copays or deductibles (the patient's required costs for care based on different plans) and therefore it can be hypothesized that many individuals do not seek preventive/wellness care, for example, annual exams for adults, breast and Pap smears for women, prostate exams for males, skin and eye evaluations, and so on. Without these interpersonal communication and relationship-building interactions between providers and patients, there is less opportunity for information sharing, collaborative decision making, and health education. As a consequence, it is more likely that patients' health/wellness will be less maintained and, as a result, will require treatment for an illness or injury with the associated higher cost of curative versus preventive care. Although the Affordable Care Act was intended to provide more access to health care, it almost certainly concomitantly encourages more interpersonal health communication exchange, education, and enhanced interpersonal relationship building, which, it is hoped, will lead to an increased health/wellness goal/attainment and reduced long-term health care costs for the nation.

Over the past 260 years, health care in America has evolved from a largely unregulated, unlicensed individual vocation, to a multicultural, diverse, inter-professional, interdependent, technologically driven, 21st-century corporate enterprise. What Benjamin Franklin could not predict when he cofounded the first U.S. hospital were the ways health care delivery and health communication would change from a predominantly single-focused doctor–patient dyadic interaction to a multiprofessional, multiorganizational, "mass communication" experience in which patients, providers, and/or organizations communicate across diverse channels (face-to-face, phone, Internet, written, electronic, etc.). For example, think of the typical hospitalized patient of today. In the course of a fairly routine 3-day stay, she or he will likely communicate, across 8- and 10-hour shifts, directly with dozens, perhaps even 100 or more health care providers:

- Doctors (MD/DO)
- RNs
  - Licensed practical nurses (LPNs)
  - Certified nursing assistants (CNAs)
  - Nurse technicians
- Midlevel providers
  - PAs
  - APRN/nurse practitioners (NPs)
  - Certified nurse-midwives (CNMs)

and many more. But these providers are likely each communicating with several other providers about the patient, including adding documentation to the patient's medical record. That written communication is then sent to the hospital's billing department, which submits it to the patient's insurance company, Medicare, or Medicaid. In addition, if there were any adverse events (complications that cause unexpected/unintended harm to the patient) that occurred during the patient's stay, then those have to be communicated to the risk-management department, perhaps to the hospital's legal staff, depending on the severity, even to the state regulatory office, and so on. And we cannot forget the patient's prescriptions being communicated to his or her pharmacy, information being sent to the patient's primary care provider (PCP) and/or specialists, and so forth. Like modern health care delivery, health communication has evolved to be equally multifaceted, interdependent, and critical to each patient's successful health outcome.

Although there is no doubt that 21st-century health care is not only highly scientific, expensive, and disease focused—it is also at its most basic totally dependent on effective interpersonal, health, intercultural, and organizational communication. And yet, as the one common denominator that crosses all health professions, interactions, diagnoses, treatments, and outcomes—communication is the one aspect of daily health care delivery that is not a *major* focus in health care provider education. The purpose of this book is to help you understand the importance of effective interpersonal, intercultural, health, and organizational communication for successful prevention, diagnosis, treatment, and wellness outcomes. It is hard to imagine anyone in 21st-century health care provider education who would suggest not teaching medical terminology. And yet what good is knowing a language (medical terminology) if you do not know how to use it effectively (with the intended audience: other providers), when/how to translate it (for patients and families), and how to communicate verbally and nonverbally using behaviors that instill trust and encourage collaboration and relationship building with others (patients, providers, organizational members, etc.). Communicating in the emotionally charged context of the 21st-century American health care system requires an understanding of the theories underlying interpersonal communication and interpersonal relationships, as well as team/organizational and intercultural communication. Armed with this knowledge you should be able to listen, assimilate, and communicate with patients, peers, and your organization more effectively. In addition, applying these theories to your health care role should help you share information, power, and decision making with patients and/or families to provide a truly collaborative health/wellness outcome.

Reflections (among the possible responses)

1.1. With so few scientific instruments at his or her disposal, what would you hypothesize would be most important to a provider's analysis of patients' diagnostic success and why?

One of the most important tools a provider has at his or her disposal for assessing a patient's health is interpersonal communication. Especially without the diagnostic tools we have today, a provider's interactions with a patient/family become even more critical. In such a situation, it would be very important to learn as much as possible about the patient's current symptoms, as well as his or her past medical as well as current social, occupational, and family histories. With basically only observation, palpation, and the provider's other senses to guide him or her, interpersonal communication and information gathering from the patient and family become critical to any efforts for a successful diagnostic and treatment outcome. However, as this book tries to highlight, these same communication needs continue to exist for 21st-century providers and, it could be argued, that with so much technology, cost, and access issues, provider–patient information exchanges are even more important.

1.2. What are three communication issues that you think contributed to the lack of standardization in health provider education from 1751 to 1900?

In general, all three are likely communication related: (a) lack of sufficient medical knowledge; (b) lack of scientific research, publication, and standardization; (c) lack of information sharing among health care providers, providers–patients, and also among health care organizations. Although there are certainly many other reasons (e.g., lack of federal/professional guidelines as well as professional and institutional licensure), these are three obvious differences between health care education/standardization then and now. It seems impossible to imagine how isolated an 18th- or 19th-century provider must have felt as she or he tried to help people with diverse diseases and injuries, many of which she or he had never seen or heard of before. Communication in health care education has clearly helped transform America's providers and delivery system.

1.3. Why might the term specialist have negative implications for patients?

Perhaps as you pondered this question you asked yourself how being classified as "special" might impact a provider's self-perception, perceived status, role, power, control, and so forth. Language is very powerful and therefore it would not be unexpected for the term *specialist* to illicit quite different perceptions from patients, peers, and other providers. We can certainly hypothesize that patients who already feel uneasy with providers because of their differences in education, experience, socioeconomic status, and so forth would feel even more uncomfortable around a "specialist." And this "dis-ease" would likely manifest itself in less patient communication, feedback, and collaboration. Research has shown that the more dissimilar Americans are from peers, the less likely we are to try to develop or maintain a relationship.

1.4. What are three reasons why technology is a major force in rising health care costs in America?

Again, this question has many possible answers, but among them surely are (a) not only is technology itself expensive (MRI machine), but in order to use it, a special room has to be constructed at an enormous price; (b) even with the cost of some technology being in the hundreds of thousands, if not millions of dollars, the competitive capitalistic system in America drives hospitals, clinics, and so on only a few miles apart to spend money for similar technology, instead of sharing the costs; (c) increased technology has resulted in increased specialization and therefore unique staff to operate equipment and specialist providers to interpret the results or utilize the technology with further increased costs (more expensive to see a specialist than a PCP). However, in addition, to the direct cost resulting from increased specialization related to technology is the indirect costs of having fewer PCPs, who are paid less money for frequently more time and work with patients and who, by definition, are not "special" providers.

1.5. If you could only afford one of the two, how would you decide between buying food for dinner and refilling your blood pressure prescription? Why?

Clearly, there is no good answer to this question and yet it is estimated that in the United States almost 20% of Americans cannot afford their prescription medications. For these patients, it is clearly a choice of food, shelter, or therapy. Although providers cannot directly impact patients' purchasing decision making, they can recognize the potential for patients, especially older Americans on a fixed income, to have financial difficulties and discuss the patient's situation and whether a different drug or generic medication might be available at a lower price to make utilization more possible. Although providers cannot change the cost of treatment, they can use interpersonal communication and their interpersonal relationship with a patient to help collaborate and find the most effective (cost and clinical) option possible and demonstrate their understanding of the patient's situation, their empathy, and the need for joint decision making.

Skills Exercise

While you are conversing with someone you know, try following up one of their statements with a series of questions, the more questions the better—even interrupting to make sure your questions get answered; try to ask them as quickly as possible. Once you are done, reflect on how it felt to be a "detective" controlling the conversation? Ask the other interactant (if she or he is still speaking to you) how it made her or him feel to suddenly be quizzed, instead of listened to, and frequently interrupted?

In a different conversation, ask a friend/classmate/loved one to tell you about his or her day, or week, and just listen until she or he finishes. Try to be conscious of your nonverbal behaviors and nod your head appropriately if you understand, or frown or make an uncertain facial gesture to show your confusion, but try very hard not to stop the other person's flow of information. When she or he is done, you should ask any questions needed to clarify and/or demonstrate your understanding of what she or he told you. When finished, think about how you felt being focused on assimilating information, not thinking about what questions you needed to get answered. Also, ask the other person what she or he noticed and/or felt about the interaction and the information she or he wanted to communicate? How do these two experiences impact your thoughts about gathering patient's information, listening versus talking, and considering the other person's needs/views in a health care setting? If you find them valuable, then why not try this latter approach to sharing information in your provider–patient interactions?

Video Discussion Exercise

Analyze the video

- *Escape Fire: The Fight to Rescue American Health* (2013)

Role-Play Using These Interactive Simulation Exercises

Pagano, M. (2015). *Communication case studies for health care professionals: An applied approach* (2nd ed.). New York, NY: Springer Publishing Company.

- Chapter 3, "The Biomedical Model" (pp. 27–34)

Health Care Issues in the Media

Nursing shortage
http://www.nytimes.com/2015/05/28/opinion/we-need-more-nurses.html?_r=0

The costs of treating cancer
https://www.youtube.com/watch?v=zf-4E9KjgQk

Health Communication Outcomes

This chapter highlights only 265 years of health care. It is important to remember that the study of illness/injury and wellness is more than 4,000 years old. However, the vast changes in health care delivery, education, and communication in contemporary America are the focus of this text. Health care in the United States has evolved exponentially over the past 100 years in large part because of changes in provider education, health insurance, technology, specialization, pharmaceutical and medical device R&D, team versus individual approaches, and government regulations. But these unprecedented scientific, clinical, and pedagogical advancements have further heightened an illness/injury focus and accompanying economic issues. The costs of health care delivery in 21st-century America is both a driving economic force (diverse employment opportunities, highly profitable health care organizations, etc.), but simultaneously a potential budget-buster for individuals, corporations, and the U.S. government. The focus on disease/injury processes, diagnosis, and treatment creates a self-perpetuating system that not only relies on illnesses and injuries for sustainability, but rewards providers, manufacturers, and health care organizations for treatment, not prevention. As long as American health care is focused on diseases/injuries and their cures, not patients, the easier it is to minimize the need for effective provider–patient communication.

■ REFERENCE

Franklin, B. (1754). *Some account of the Pennsylvania hospital: From its first rise to the beginning.* Philadelphia, PA: Franklin & Hall.

■ BIBLIOGRAPHY

Congress Blog. (2014, November 12). Americans can't afford U.S. medication, need a safe alternative. *The Hill*. Retrieved from http://thehill.com/blogs/congress-blog/healthcare/223650-americans-cant-afford-us-medication-need-a-safe-alternative

Foucault, M. (1973). *The birth of the clinic: An archaeology of medical perception* (pp. 107–123). New York, NY: Vintage.

Goldsteen, R., & Goldsteen, K. (2013). *Jonas' introduction to the U.S. Health Care System* (7th ed., pp. 75–117). New York, NY: Springer Publishing Company.

HHS.gov/HealthCare. (2014). *Affordable Care Act: About the law*. Retrieved from http://www.hhs.gov/healthcare/rights

Kohn, L., Corrigan, J., & Donaldson, M. (Eds.). (2000). *To err is human: Building a safer health system*. Washington, DC: National Academies Press.

MediLexicon. (2014). *Full FDA prescription drug list*. Retrieved from http://www.medilexicon.com/drugsearch.php?z=true

Organisation for Economic Co-operation and Development. (2011). *Society at a glance 2011: OECD social indicators* (6th ed.). Paris, France: OECD Publishing. doi:10.1787/soc_glance-2011-en

Shi, L., & Singh, D. (2013). *Essentials of the U.S. health care system* (3rd ed., pp. 1–29). Sudbury, MA: Jones & Bartlett.

Starr, P. (1982). *The social transformation of American medicine: The rise of a sovereign profession and the making of a vast industry*. New York, NY: Basic Books.

Sultz, H., & Young, K. (2006). *Health care USA: Understanding its organization and delivery* (5th ed.). Sudbury, MA: Jones & Bartlett.

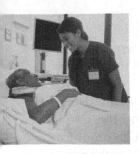

CHAPTER 2

Health Care Pedagogy

For the purpose of this text, we are going to use the following as working definitions:

- *Apprentice:* Learning a skill or trade from someone, not necessarily requiring any formal classroom training
- *Artifacts:* Clothing, hair styles, make-up, beards, jewelry, tattoos, piercings, and so forth
- *Culture:* The beliefs, values, goals, language, and so forth of a group of people (e.g., a country, the United States; or an organization, American Nursing Association or American Medical Association)
- *Coculture:* The beliefs, values, goals, language, and so forth of a group of people within a larger culture (e.g., nurses, doctors, hospital administrators)
- *Discipline:* Profession (e.g., doctor, nurse) or specialty within a profession (obstetrics, radiology, surgery)
- *Interdiscipline:* Across professions (e.g., doctors and nurses)
- *Intradiscipline:* Within the same profession (e.g., among doctors or between nurses)

■ HEALTH COMMUNICATION: A GENERALIST APPROACH

As pointed out in Chapter 1, this text takes a generalist view of health communication. Therefore, we will be exploring all aspects of American health care and its impact on a wide variety of health communication contexts and audiences. This diverse discussion will include how health care delivery is taught to providers, how disease and wellness are communicated to patients, how providers share information with each other (intra- and interprofessionally), and how health care organizations disseminate messages to members, stakeholders, and/or customers/clients/patients. However, the impact of the federal government, laws (national and state), and regulations will also be important to our understanding of U.S. health care delivery and the role of communication. Therefore, let's begin our exploration of health communication by considering the role health provider pedagogy plays in the exchange of information and its impact on patient care and outcomes.

Reflection 2.1. In what ways (positively and negatively) do you think provider education impacts provider–patient and provider–provider communication?

_____

_____

_____

_____

_____

■ TRAINING PROVIDERS: THE EARLY YEARS

As discussed in Chapter 1, prior to 1910 health care providers in the United States were trained through highly unregulated, disjointed approaches, predominantly as apprentices. While some providers did attend medical and nursing schools during this period, even those who did were not receiving any standardized education across institutions. Some medical schools, for example, included laboratory study, others did not, textbooks were not standardized or peer reviewed and, during this time, there were no formal state or federal regulations for opening or operating a professional school. In short, nearly anyone who wanted to create a medical or nursing school could do so and provide students with a degree/certificate upon completion.

As mentioned, many health care providers in the 18th and 19th centuries did not attend a professional school, but instead apprenticed with a practicing provider. As a consequence, new doctors, nurses, and so forth, were only as well educated as the mentor with whom he or she was apprenticing and the mistakes, misperceptions, miscommunications, and misinformation of one provider was passed on to the next. Although it can be argued that 21st-century health care still uses a form of apprenticeship in educating modern providers, vis-à-vis clinical training in professional schools, postgraduate residencies, and fellowships—the differences between the first 150-plus years of health care education in America and the most recent 100 years can be traced in large part to the involvement and regulation of the U.S. government.

Reflection 2.2. How do you think learning to be a health provider only in a classroom setting, or only training one-on-one with a provider who learned in a similar fashion, might create health communication problems for providers and patients?

_____

_____

_____

_____

_____

■ TRAINING PROVIDERS: THE FLEXNER REPORT

In 1910, Abraham Flexner released his 5-year study of American professional schools, which was commissioned by the Carnegie Foundation. This was the most thorough examination of U.S. provider education at the time and it found enormous inconsistencies and problems. Specifically, the report found:

(1) For the past 25 years there has been an enormous over-production of un-educated and ill-trained medical practitioners. This has been an absolute disregard of the public welfare and without any serious thought of the interests of the public. . . . (2) Over-production of ill-trained men is due in the main to the existence of a very large number of commercial schools, sustained in many cases by advertising methods through which a mass of unprepared youth is drawn out of industrial occupations into the study of medicine. (3) Until recently the conduct of a medical school was a profitable business, for the methods of instruction were mainly didactic. As the need for laboratories has become more keenly felt, the expenses of an efficient medical school have been greatly increased. . . . (4) The existence of many of these unnecessary and inadequate medical schools has been defended by the argument that a poor medical school is justified in the interest of the poor boy. It is clear that the poor boy has no right to go into any profession for which he is not willing to obtain adequate preparation; but the facts set forth in this report make it evident that this argument is insincere, and that the excuse which has hitherto been put forward in the name of the poor boy is in reality an argument in behalf of the poor medical school. (5) A hospital under complete educational control is as necessary to a medical school as is a laboratory of chemistry or pathology. High grade teaching within a hospital introduces a most wholesome and beneficial influence into its routine. Trustees of hospitals, public and private, should therefore go to the limit of their authority in opening hospital

wards to teaching, provided only that the universities secure sufficient funds on their side to employ as teachers men who are devoted to clinical science. (Introduction, para. 16)

The Flexner Report illustrates the frightening realities of pre-20th-century American medical education and health care delivery. Not only was there an overabundance of medical training facilities, but these institutions were unregulated and not educating their students effectively and the results were at a minimum dangerous and at worst deadly. Clearly, the report highlighted several health communication issues, among them the need to properly educate future providers, but also the need to evolve beyond just didactic teaching to include laboratory experiences, research, and clinical skills, as well as apprentice-like education in a hospital that was controlled by a medical school using teachers who were interested in clinical science. This awareness of the communication and health care delivery problems created by uneven or inept pedagogy and the impact on patient care is critical to our understanding of what transpired following this report.

Reflection 2.3. Why would the Flexner Report stress laboratory studies and work in a medical school–controlled hospital as being important criteria for future medical education?

_____

_____

_____

_____

_____

■ BIOMEDICAL MODEL

Effective health communication and health care delivery are ultimately dependent upon properly educated providers. Without up-to-date scientific and clinical knowledge, providers could not be expected to assist patients in overcoming illness, injury, and/or maintaining wellness. Consequently, there can be little doubt as to the critical importance of health communication to health care pedagogy and ultimately to successful diagnosis and treatment, but also to effective information sharing, collaborative decision making, and desired health outcomes. One of the major goals of the post–Flexner Report era was the development of a health care culture that included a scientific approach to both the study and practice of patient care.

This new physician coculture sought to exemplify the role of the physician as an expert—based on advanced scientific and clinical education.

This notion of a doctor as an expert was very important in overcoming the educational shortcomings and problems identified in the Flexner Report. By making medical education more standardized and rigorous, with licensure the norm, the coculture intended to verbally and nonverbally change patients' perceptions of the profession. Furthermore, this new coculture would be based on goals like combating illness and injury, as well as increasing life expectancy and enhancing health outcomes. Accomplishing these goals would require a unique language of medical terminology, and prescribed values based on the Hippocratic Oath. Members of this coculture would be expected to dress differently than the larger culture, usually in a white coat (short for students, long for faculty/providers), professional attire, or scrub clothes (later in the century). From a communication perspective, it is important to recognize how, over the next 100 years, these cultural decisions helped to visually and verbally elevate the role of physician from an everyman to a unique, highly educated expert. The more the coculture worked to personify the status, role, and education of physicians as clinical scientists, the more the larger culture began to perceive them as irreplaceable professionals and community leaders. American society's recognition of the need for highly trained and licensed physicians was one of the catalysts for medical schools to illustrate how doctors were being trained to identify and treat illnesses and injuries, as well as develop and operate ever-advancing health care technologies.

Charged with expanding the health care knowledge as well as the scientific and clinical skills of post–Flexner Report medical students, it seems logical that medical education would focus on identifying and treating diseases and injuries. From a communication perspective it makes sense that providers would need to first research and examine the etiology of a disease in order to find a way to cure it. Therefore, a biomedical approach to medical education was chosen as the ideal way to highlight the biological aspects of illness and injury. Physicians learned how to identify various anatomical, physiological, and biological problems and the appropriate medical and surgical treatment options required to treat each. This focus on disease and injury relied on the use of a provider's mechanistic lens to first identify a problem with the human body and then find a way to fix it. Metaphorically conceiving of the body as complex collection of machine-like parts (the heart as a pump, the lymph nodes as filters, the brain as a control panel, etc.) allowed medical education to focus on teaching students about the parts (anatomy), how they work (physiology), how they become damaged (clinical medicine/surgery), and how to fix them (pharmacology/surgery). From a health communication/pedagogical perspective it made great sense to take a mechanistic approach to the study of medicine, because it allowed students to focus on diseases and their treatments. In addition, the biomedical approach not only supported the need for technological advances to better understand the "machine," but required the development of diverse specialized tools for use in diagnosis, research, and treatment.

Reflection 2.4. If you were a provider using a biomedical model, how would you use communication (what kinds of questions would you ask) with a patient to identify a problem?

_____

_____

_____

_____

■ BIOMEDICAL, TECHNOLOGICAL SPECIALIZATION

As medical education increasingly focused on the biomedical aspects of health, it became clear that new and/or improved technologies would be needed to help further research and understand human anatomy, physiology, microbiology, and so forth. With each new or enhanced technological advancement, it became increasingly important to have providers who focused on how best to utilize and interpret the results of a particular test or treatment modality. Therefore, technology and the biomedical focus of medical education led to the need for provider specialization.

Specialists, who could have been perceived as narrowly focused providers who were not as expert as general practitioners, by their very title, became recognized as "special" doctors. It seems odd that a general/family physician who treats children, adults, even does surgery, was frequently perceived as less knowledgeable and skilled than specialists. In addition, the generalists who provide the gatekeeping—determining who needs to see a specialist—as well as the highly valued continuity of care for patients—are all paid less than specialists. As a consequence, with the increased status (cardiovascular and neurological surgeons vs. general surgeons, pulmonologists and pathologists vs. family physicians), the more specialized a provider is, generally, the more he or she uses technology and the narrower is his or her disease/anatomic focus. As more technologies for a particular anatomic/physiologic structure/process were created (e.g., EKG, stress tests, cardiac catheterization, stents), the more providers became specialists (e.g., cardiologists and cardiovascular surgeons). This parallel rise in technology and specialization had a direct impact on patient care and health care delivery. The increasing status, roles, and income for specialists mirrored the rising value of technological benefits for diagnosis and treatment regimens. Unfortunately for U.S. health care, the concomitant rise in specialization and technology led to a decrease in medical students becoming general/family practice physicians and a huge increase in health-related costs. Specialists, by their very title, are paid more than nonspecialists and with each new advance in technology, there is almost always an increase in cost. And, as discussed previously, many of these are more than just direct costs ($1 million for a machine), but indirect costs, like $500,000 for a new room to house the machine, $10,000 for additional electricity to power it, plus more money for a specialist technician who operates it, and so forth. Although this marked increase in specialization, technology, and health care costs over the past 100 years has directly impacted health communication (more difficult for patients to communicate with a specialist and less power/control sharing) and health care delivery (especially access to care and costs), not all cocultures focus on a biomedical approach to health care pedagogy.

Reflection 2.5. You are a board-certified specialist. Who then should be making a patient's treatment decisions: You? The patient? Both of you? Why?

_____

_____

_____

_____

_____

■ THE NURSING COCULTURE

It is impossible to talk about health care provider pedagogy without discussing nursing's approach to this important topic. Prior to the 20th century, nurses were primarily trained in hospitals. However, after the Flexner Report, even though nursing was not its focus, the coculture of nursing became more education oriented, standardized, and licensed. Furthermore, nursing pedagogy evolved from being predominantly hospital-based training, to a 2-year associate degree education, and, in the latter half of the 20th century, to a 4-year bachelor's degree. Like medicine, the coculture of nursing has its own values, but these are more patient centric than medical schools and included goals that focused more on patients' health than just disease identification. The nursing coculture had its own artifacts, frequently a white dress and cap, which later evolved to pants, or scrub clothes, or professional business-styled attire. Nursing coculture also shares the same language/terminology as physicians. However, nursing pedagogy is based on a significantly different philosophical system than medicine—the biopsychosocial approach.

■ BIOPSYCHOSOCIAL MODEL

As the biomedical model of the medicine coculture is disease centric and uses a find-it, fix-it, mechanistic approach to health care diagnosis and treatment, nursing pedagogy adopted a more patient-focused, biopsychosocial model that communicated to the members of its culture and the larger U.S. culture that although there are biological causes for illness, there are also psychological and sociological etiologies and/or contributing factors to a patient's illness, injury, or wellness. This seemingly philosophical/pedagogical distinction is also a significant health communication statement to patients and families. By its very nature, an approach to health care that recognizes emotional and social influences moves beyond disease and injury to an awareness of the complex and multifocal nature of human existence, health, and wellness.

Consider, from a health communication perspective, what it means to approach a patient with a "find-it, fix-it," provider-focused, mechanistic lens versus a "tell me how you are feeling" patient-centered, interpersonal relationship-building (two people sharing information and similar goals) approach. Both medicine and nursing pedagogies emphasize scientific and clinical inquiry, experience, and expertise; however, the nursing coculture vis-à-vis a biopsychosocial approach communicates its belief in exploring health, not just disease, and doing so from a patient's perspective. It should be pointed out, however, that using a more patient-centered model has not precluded nursing from being part of the specialized approach to 21st-century health care delivery. Nurses generally are employed in specialty areas, like labor and delivery, or surgery, or emergency departments. However, unlike physicians who tend to specialize in these areas, nurses, perhaps in part because of their patient-focused approach, are able much more easily to move from one specialty area to another. For physician specialists, the need to commit 3 to 6 years of residency training in a specialty, along with having to pass a specialty board examination, makes it very difficult to change specialties. These differences in health care pedagogies and philosophies contribute to some of the intercultural issues in contemporary American health care delivery.

Reflection 2.6. Using a biopsychosocial approach to health communication, how would you inquire about the reason for a patient's visit to your clinic or office?

_____

_____

_____

_____

_____

■ THE CULTURE OF HEALTH CARE

This chapter has focused on health care pedagogy and how it is impacted by and/or alters health communication and health care delivery. We've discussed the various ways medicine and nursing cocultures can be identified and categorized, through their artifacts, goals, communication behaviors, education, and so forth. However, 21st-century U.S. health care is much more interdependent, intercultural, and team organized. Therefore, effective health communication in contemporary health care delivery is more critically important to successful patient outcomes than ever before. In an age of expanding technology and specialization, effective patient–provider, provider–provider, and health care organizational communication are crucial to attaining common goals—patient health/wellness, decreased risks/adverse events, and decreased health care costs.

The reality that nursing and medicine cocultures share two languages (U.S. English and medical/nursing terminology), common goals (patient health/wellness, decreased risks/adverse events), and values (not to harm patients and improve quality of care) are some of the reasons why health care is as productive and effective as it is in America today. However, other aspects of the disparities between nursing and physician cocultures (language/literacy, power, control, etc.) contribute to our current U.S. health care delivery problems. With fewer general/family practice providers to assess and triage patients and a continued focus on disease/injury instead of health/wellness, there are added burdens placed on emergency departments, lack of continuity of care, and decreased patient trust and too often limited compliance. In order to further explore the current health care delivery issues in this country, but also examine how they may be more effectively addressed—the next chapter describes the potential impact of interpersonal and gendered communication on providers' and patients' interactions, collaborations, and decision making.

Reflections (among the possible responses)

2.1. In what ways (positively and negatively) do you think provider education impacts provider–patient and provider–provider communication?

Clearly, provider education has an enormous impact on provider–patient and provider–provider communication as both rely on the effective exchange of information. However, to truly share information and/or assess various data, providers must fully analyze both the material and the audience. Consequently, knowing something and being able to apply that knowledge effectively, as well as being able to communicate it in a way that a receiver (patient, family, peer, etc.) can assimilate and utilize it are not inevitabilities. Provider education strives to assure that health professionals have the information needed to diagnose and treat patients. Provider education also uses exams and clinical work to help providers demonstrate their abilities, regardless of their profession, to apply the knowledge they have assimilated from their didactic and clinical studies in patient care. However, few health professional education programs offer much if any specific theoretical and applied courses in, or assessments of, student–provider's health communication.

2.2. How do you think learning to be a health provider only in a classroom setting, or only training one-on-one with a provider who learned in a similar fashion, might create health communication problems for providers and patients?

One of the major flaws with an apprenticeship approach to education is that the student is limited in his or her learning by the knowledge base and teaching ability of the mentor. Therefore a single physician who is the sole source of education for a student, regardless of how much he or she knows, could only hope to communicate that limited information. Similarly, only having a didactic education eliminates the student's opportunities to apply that knowledge in an educational environment where mistakes can be caught and corrected with minimal pain for patients and/or negative outcomes (residencies versus role-play/simulation). The goal of contemporary professional education is to expose health care students to a breadth of ideas, professors, approaches, knowledge, and experience. Similarly, students learning from multiple faculty in didactic and clinical situations are also offered the opportunity to learn from their various professors' communication behaviors and adapt their verbal and nonverbal behaviors based on their assessment of what will be the most effective in a given context (e.g., birth of a healthy baby versus birth of a baby with a congenital defect, or the diagnosis of a malignancy, or a terminal illness). However, without formal communication courses students are left to decide on their own which behaviors are effective and which are not. The problem for many provider–patient interactions is often not the science, but the communication of that science.

2.3. Why would the Flexner Report stress laboratory studies and work in a medical school–controlled hospital as being important criteria for future medical education?

Credibility is an important quality, especially for providers who need patients to trust their knowledge, skills, and judgment. However, the Flexner Report (Flexner, 1910) highlighted the country's problems with many poorly educated physicians. Therefore, in order to overcome patients' possible perceptions that American health care delivery could not be trusted, the report stressed visual and objective ways to demonstrate to future patients that their health care providers were being competently educated, challenged, and critiqued in both didactic and clinical situations. Persuasion relies on effective communication in order to change perceptions and ultimately behaviors. The Flexner Report recognized the need to persuade Americans that their health care delivery system was providing a rigorous, comprehensive, consistent, and critically assessed provider education. By establishing the breadth and depth of a provider's training (didactic and clinical), it would seem that patients could be expected to recognize their providers as experts and more likely to trust their analyses and recommendations.

2.4. If you were a provider using a biomedical model, how would you use communication (what kinds of questions would you ask) with a patient to identify a problem?

Because the biomedical model relies on identifying a problem, it would be expected that a provider's queries about a patient's concern would be focused on determining first what are the patient's signs (objective, anyone can see them: fever, rash, hemoptysis [blood in sputum] and symptoms; subjective, only the patient is aware of them: pain, dizziness, parasthesias [tingling in an arm or leg]). Therefore, it would make the most sense to ask closed-ended questions in order to gain the data the provider needs for his or her assessment (e.g.,"do you have a fever, blood in your sputum, a rash?"). Or to inquire about stated symptoms, when closed-ended questions would help to focus the patient's responses to the specific anatomical or physiological processes that the provider is interested in assessing (e.g.,"where is your rash, when did it start, have you had it before, do you have any allergies?"). The use of closed-ended questions (yes, or no, or very specific answers are expected, e.g., "my fever was 102.4 degrees last night.") helps both the patient and the provider focus on the disease/injury and discourages discussion of other issues that the patient might otherwise want to raise (e.g., emotional and/or social). Under the biomedical model, the provider, not the patient, controls the interaction, the information requested, and the determination of when to close/end the conversation. Not unlike when we take a car to a mechanic, he or she is the expert and is expected to find the problem and fix it. However, unlike our cars, contemporary Americans are more educated than ever before and many want to better understand not just the treatment prescribed, but the findings, analysis, and possible alternate treatment options. From a health communication perspective, using a biomedical model, does not generally fit with a collaborative, participative view of health care delivery and shared decision making.

2.5. You are a board-certified specialist. Who then should be making a patient's treatment decisions: You? The patient? Both of you? Why?

This question is philosophical, but also extremely relevant. Although it is true that health care specialists generally have more knowledge than patients, this reality does not necessarily mean the specialist should be making decisions for patients. Contractors, financial advisers, lawyers, and so forth are all experts and yet most Americans want to gather information from these professionals, analyze it, and then collaborate with the expert to arrive at the best decision for them and/or their families. Therefore, health care, which is generally one of the most highly emotionally charged contexts that humans communicate in, could be expected to encourage more collaborations than construction, finance, and so forth. However, specialists, by the very nature of that title, often see themselves as so knowledgeable that their decisions, prescriptions, plans, should not be discussed, let alone questioned. If patients are to truly trust their providers it would seem that building an interpersonal relationship through information sharing and disclosure, equalizing power, and working collaboratively would be the most effective way to accomplish the common goal of enhanced patient health/wellness/quality of life.

2.6. Using a biopsychosocial approach to health communication, how would you inquire about the reason for a patient's visit to your clinic or office?

As opposed to using a biomedical model to focus a health communication interaction, a biopsychosocial approach would expect a provider to use open-ended, not closed-ended, questions to generate more data and a more traditional interpersonal communication exchange. For example, a provider using a biopsychosocial style might initiate a conversation with a patient by asking, "tell me how you're doing?" or "what's going on?" These very abstract, conversational queries would be intended to allow the patient to tell his or her health story (narrative). Using open-ended questions at the outset of an interaction allows the patient to manage the information sharing and helps to equalize the control and power between the provider and the patient. As the provider listens, rather than talks, he or she is able to gather data related to the patient's biological, psychological, and sociological condition and then the provider can use more closed-ended queries to gather more specific details: signs, symptoms, concerns, and so forth. In American culture, we are by nature storytellers and therefore providing patients an opportunity to tell their health/illness stories can be expected to encourage not only information sharing, but relationship building, trust, and collaboration.

Skills Exercise

Think back to your last provider interaction in which you were the patient, what do you recall of the provider's communication skills? Did he or she encourage you to discuss the reason(s) why you were there? Did the provider stand over you, or sit at your eye level? How did the provider's communication make you feel about the experience? Now think of a time when you went to a counselor (professional or religious), friend, and/or loved one to discuss a problem. How were your perceptions of the two conversations—from communication behaviors, information sharing, and trust—altered by the person's verbal and nonverbal behaviors? How can you use this analysis in your efforts to be a more effective health care provider/communicator?

Video Discussion Exercise

Analyze the video

- *Awakenings* (1990)

Interactive Simulation Exercise

Pagano, M. (2015). *Communication case studies for health care professionals: An applied approach* (2nd ed.). New York, NY: Springer Publishing Company.

- Chapter 1, "Learning to Talk Like a Health Care Provider" (pp. 5–16)
- Chapter 2, "See One, Do One, Teach One" (pp. 17–26)
- Chapter 4, "The Biopsychosocial Model" (pp. 35–44)

Health Care Issues in the Media

Doctors in training
http://www.nytimes.com/2009/03/03/health/03zion.html

Clinical simulation training
http://www.nytimes.com/1999/10/28/technology/wired-virtual-patients-simulate-emergencies-for-students.html

Health Communication Outcomes

For more than 150 years, health care provider education in America was based on unregulated programs and/or apprentice-style training before it completely changed with the Industrial Revolution. Based on the Flexner Report and other influences, health care pedagogy became not only regulated, but also organized, more science based, and clinically focused. However, with an objective-, research-, data-driven approach to health care, patient–provider communication took on a similar style. With the emphasis on disease identification and evidence-based treatment, providers became more like detectives and researchers than collaborators and educators. The biomedical model was developed to assure a scientific approach to health care delivery, however, this find-it, fix-it mentality left little room for patient participation, nurturing, and interpersonal relationship development. Providers, especially physicians, became experts at diagnosis and treatment, but frequently relied more on a paternalistic, authoritarian communication style in order to get the information needed in a format that worked best for the provider/researcher/detective. Nursing pedagogy took a different path and, although it recognized the importance of assessing the biological etiologies of illnesses and injuries, it was also acutely focused on how a patient's psychological and sociological situations could impact the patient's health and wellness. Throughout the 20th century, this biopsychosocial view of health/wellness has led to an understanding of the importance of quality-of-life assessment and prognosis for patients and their families. In consequence, as the biomedical model focuses more on the information needs of the provider, the biopsychosocial approach is patient centric and relies more on narratives, open-ended queries, information sharing, and interpersonal communication and relationship development. Throughout the 20th century, the art and science as well as the culture of health care have been rapidly evolving; however, for the most part it has remained a provider-centric, disease-focused exploration and provider–patient communication is frequently viewed as a tool for scientific discovery rather than a concomitant opportunity to share information, build trust, develop relationships, and enhance collaborative decision making.

■ REFERENCE

Flexner, A. (1910). *Medical education in the United States and Canada: A report to the Carnegie Foundation for the advancement of teaching.* Retrieved from http://archive.org/stream/medicaleducation00flexiala/medicaleducation00flexiala_djvu.txt

■ BIBLIOGRAPHY

Association of American Physicians and Surgeons. (2014). *The Oath of Hippocrates of Kos, 5th century BC.* Retrieved from http://www.aapsonline.org/ethics/oaths.htm

Duffy, R. (2011). The Flexner Report—100 years later. *Yale Journal of Biology and Medicine, 84*(3), 269–276.

Klainberg, M., & Kirschel, K. (2009). *Today's nursing leader: Managing, succeeding, excelling.* Sudbury, MA: Jones & Bartlett.

Krupa, C. (2010, October 4). Medical education still evolving 100 years after Flexner Report. *American Medical News.* Retrieved from http://www.amednews.com/article/20101004/profession/310049932/7

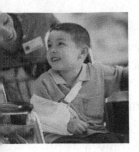

CHAPTER 3

Interpersonal and Gendered Communication

For the purpose of this text, we are going to use the following as working definitions:

- *Communication competence:* the ability to effectively exchange and process information with others

- *Context:* setting or situation

- *Empathic listening:* letting speakers talk without interruption and demonstrating the listener's support without evaluating the speaker or providing instruction, instead encouraging the speaker to find a solution

- *Feedback:* using statements or questions to demonstrate listening to a sender or to encourage clarification from a receiver

- *Gender:* gender may not be constant or easily determined by others and is different from a person's sex; it is demonstrated by how an individual chooses to behave/act, that is, masculine, feminine, or more likely somewhere in between

- *Gender identity:* a person's perception of his or her masculinity or femininity

- *Goal competence:* the capability to construct goals and choose a plan(s) to accomplish them

- *Interpersonal (also known as dyadic) communication:* interactions between two people *who know each other and share common goals* (e.g., friends, lovers, family members, professionals, and a provider and a patient); it is not the same as an infrequent conversation between a customer and a store clerk or a restaurant waitperson

- *Interpersonal relationship:* a bond between two people who share common goals requiring effective interpersonal communication for its development and/or maintainenance

- *Nonverbal communication:* behaviors that are not word based; messages transmitted via observable or experienced actions (eye contact, touch, vocal volume, tone, etc.)

- *Role competence:* the skill to assume various social/professional roles based on the context and communicators' goals

- *Self-disclosure:* sharing highly personal information with only a very limited number of most intimate friends/lovers

- *Sex:* male or female, generally anatomically obvious to self and others; determined by presence of a vagina in a female or a penis in a male

- *Verbal communication:* literally what you hear or say when in a conversation with one or more interactants

■ INTERPERSONAL COMMUNICATION AND HEALTH CARE

As you may have surmised from the aforementioned definitions, interpersonal communication is critical to our interactions with friends, family, and lovers, but it is also vital to successful outcomes in our professional lives. Perhaps no profession depends on the effective use of interpersonal communication exchanges more than health care. If you spend a minute to think of a recent visit to your own health care provider, or an interaction you had with a patient, you will likely understand that at the most basic level, almost all health communication is interpersonal. Health care providers and patients are constantly engaging in information sharing to assure effective diagnosis, testing, treatment, and outcomes. But just as critical is the interpersonal communication between health care providers. Regardless of the channel (air waves, electronic, written, etc.), and whether it is verbal or nonverbal, providers needs to share information with other providers (intra- and interprofessionally) in order to achieve their patient goals, minimize risk, and attain successful outcomes.

Reflection 3.1. Thinking about a single interaction (with your provider, a colleague provider, or with a patient), how would you describe the communication exchange? Was it effective or problematic and why?

_____

_____

_____

_____

_____

Understanding the role of interpersonal communication in health care is critical to the focus of this book. Once we recognize that almost all of our health care interactions are interpersonal, the value of understanding the theories and skills needed to be an effective communicator becomes glaringly obvious. And with that reality comes the recognition that for two people who share common goals (a patient's health), the importance of developing and maintaining an interpersonal relationship becomes even more paramount. As we know from our personal lives, those friends, family members, lovers, and colleagues, with whom we have an interpersonal relationship are generally the people whom we trust, share information with, and value the most. Therefore, as a health care provider you will benefit greatly if you can strive to develop an interpersonal relationship with your patients, as well as your peers, colleagues, and superiors.

However, we cannot hope to accomplish effective interpersonal health communication and relationship development without a clear understanding of the impact of gendered behaviors on information exchanges, trust, collaboration, and goal planning/attainment. Therefore, this chapter explores how interpersonal and gendered communication in health care are so important to interpersonal relationship development and maintenance. And, as previously mentioned, in this culture we tend to share information more fully, listen to, collaborate with, and trust those with whom we have an effective interpersonal relationship.

Reflection 3.2. Can you recall a situation in which you needed help from someone, or that person offered advice about something? Did/would your reactions to that offer change based on an interpersonal relationship with that person? If so, why? If not, why not?

_____

_____

_____

_____

_____

■ BUILDING RELATIONSHIPS

For the purpose of this text, we are discussing professional relationships (provider–patient, provider–provider, provider–family member, etc.). As you know from your own relationships, they generally begin when one person becomes aware of another; in health care contexts, this may be the first time a patient goes to a provider, or the first time a provider begins working with another provider, and so forth. Based on the interpersonal communication of that initial contact, as well as the circumstances (patient's wellness/illness, health care team, etc.), interactants will make decisions about the other person and future contact/communication. We need to constantly remind ourselves how different health care, as a profession/context, is from other areas of our lives. For example, we tend to have lots of everyday relationships. Some illustrations of these affiliations are the barista at the local coffee shop or the salesperson at the clothing store. While it may be nice to see a familiar face each time you visit, you will likely not change your behaviors if there is someone else who replaces him or her. And although the person in these everyday roles may be friendly, remember your name, clothing size, drink order, and so forth, you do not share common goals. These everyday relationships generally revolve around your desire/need for something versus the other person's goal to sell something, keep his or her job, or influence the boss. As you can see, for most health care professionals, this is not the type of relationship that makes sense if you are trying to gather/share information. And while health care employees certainly want to keep their jobs and impress their superiors, generally speaking their primary goal is to help patients maintain or reestablish their wellness and achieve the best quality of life possible—which are almost always patients' goals as well.

Based on this understanding of an interpersonal relationship with shared goal(s), provider–patient and provider–provider interactions need to have some common understandings:

1. There are expectations that each interactant agrees to adhere to
2. Rules are needed to assure both confidentiality and privacy, as well as trust and openness
3. An understanding that both provider and patient must be willing to do the work of not only maintaining the relationship, but attaining the shared goal(s)

In order for the relationship to develop and be most effective, both providers and patients have a right to expect that the information shared is accurate, complete, and effectively communicated. Therefore, if the patient refuses to discuss his or her prior drug use, it needs to be understood that the provider's decisions, recommendations, and so forth may not be as effective as they would have been if the patient had been more communicative. Similarly, if the provider knows about risks or alternative outcomes, she or he would be expected to share those with the patient. One of the often nonverbalized rules in provider–patient health communication includes the need for patients to fully disclose their present, past, family, and social histories, but providers will not reciprocate. Another rule is that providers will not allow a conflict of interest (financial or professional) to negatively impact the patient's care, wellness, or quality of life. Finally, the patient has a right to expect that the provider is not only qualified to offer care, but uses continuing education to update knowledge, decision making, information sharing, and so forth.

Now that we have discussed some of the important aspects of developing and maintaining an interpersonal relationship in a health care context, we need to explore the communication competencies needed to help providers effectively exchange information, enhance trust, and encourage collaborative decision making with other interactants.

Reflection 3.3. If you are in a relationship (platonic or romantic) and the other person self-discloses something very personal, what do you think that person expects in return? Why would that reality make it even harder for patients to self-disclose to providers?

_____

_____

_____

_____

_____

■ VERBAL AND NONVERBAL COMPETENCIES

Verbal Communication

As you can imagine, being an effective interpersonal communicator relies on your verbal and nonverbal competencies. Let us first focus, however, on your understanding of verbal communication. It may seem like commonsense, but when we refer to verbal behaviors we are literally discussing the use of spoken symbols (language) to exchange information. The problem for many health care professionals is the difference in their perception of shared symbols and the reality for their patients and/or family members. We discuss the culture of health care in more detail in Chapter 5, but it helps if we recognize that providers are assimilated into the health care culture (nursing, medicine, physician assistant, physical therapy, etc.) in part by learning a new shared language—medical terminology.

Because most health care providers have a bachelor's degree at a minimum, their literacy level is already advanced beyond that of the average American. To further understand the problem, we should examine some statistics from U.S. Department of Education, National Institute of Literacy (2015) regarding adult Americans:

- More than 30,000,000 cannot read
- Nearly 50% cannot understand prescription labels
- Nearly 50% are unable to read an eighth-grade-level book
- Nearly 20% of high school graduates cannot read

Although these numbers seem difficult to comprehend, they have remained relatively unchanged for decades (U.S. Department of Education, National Center for Education Statistics, 2015). Therefore, based on these data, there is a high likelihood that many of your patients will have extremely low literacy levels and have difficulty even with everyday American English. As a consequence, health communication becomes even more problematic—patients have limited literacy and providers typically use terminology that is not even remotely part of the patient's or family members' vernacular.

The first step then in understanding verbal competency for a health care provider is to recognize the role symbol sharing plays in effective communication. Next, it is critical to recognize the importance of context in communication exchanges. Perhaps if you think about a typical dinner with your family—in that context you communicate verbally using symbols that you know are most appropriate for such an audience. Suppose you go from dinner with your family, to a bar/club to relax with your friends, will your use of language/symbols change with the context? If you are like most Americans they will. Now what do you think will happen to your use of symbols when you enter a professional context? Again, they will likely change, perhaps drastically. As a health care provider, you will need to use the appropriate language/terminology with colleagues and superiors, which requires symbols that are far different than those at your family dinner or your evening out with friends. Like many Americans, you will be able to subconsciously alter your symbol usage based on the context. However, health care is unlike almost any other context because providers must use the appropriate symbols/terminology with their peers and colleagues and a very different level of symbol sharing with patients and family members.

Reflection 3.4. Besides literacy, what do you think is another major obstacle in the health care context for effective interpersonal communication and information exchange?

_____

_____

_____

_____

_____

When we think about the differences in health care communication and most other contexts, one major problem seems to transcend all others—patients' emotional responses. In the current health care system, we tend to have an acute versus chronic care focus—both as providers and as patients. For the most part, adults are not seeking care unless they have a problem. Consequently, patients come to most health interactions with verbalized, or often nonverbalized, concerns (e.g., quality of life, financial implications, pain, survival). These emotional issues may add an additional layer of difficulty to the provider–patient interaction.

Imagine if you will that you find a lump in your breast—male or female—what is likely the first thing you may assume that lump represents? Even if you are a seasoned health care provider, you are likely to be concerned that you could have cancer. Now, try to consider what it would be like not to be a health care provider with your knowledge of statistics for breast lumps for people of your age group and sex. Patients not only may be terrified that they have cancer, but some may be so concerned that they do not seek care immediately—too afraid to even tell anyone about it. Others may seek care, but not want to disclose all the information the provider is seeking in fear that by talking about a positive family history, or other potential signs and symptoms, they will increase the chances that the lump is malignant. Therefore, one thing that the emotions associated with many health care contexts contribute to provider–patient interactions is a level of "noise" that jeopardizes effective interpersonal communication and relationship development. Noise in this case is hindering the conveyance of information that providers need to help accurately assess the problem/situation. However, emotional issues in health care contexts create another type of noise that can be just as problematic for patients and providers—if not more so.

Reflection 3.5. Can you recall an exam or a lecture during which you had trouble concentrating because of something that had happened in your life? What was causing your distraction (a breakup with a lover, a death of a loved one, other unexpected joyous or sad news)?

_____

_____

_____

_____

_____

Another example of noise that interferes with effective information exchanges is the emotional concerns that distract a patient (or a provider) and decrease his or her ability to listen and assimilate what is being communicated. Think about your response to Reflection 3.5; haven't we all experienced distractions from outside events that made it very difficult to concentrate on what was happening in the present? Even if you cannot recall such a situation, you likely can understand how the death of a loved one, for example, might make it difficult to focus on a lecture, an exam, or a workplace assignment. Therefore, you should be able to see how a patient who thinks she or he has a serious illness, terminal condition, requires surgery, can no longer work, and so forth, would have a great deal of difficulty listening effectively to a provider who was trying to explain something, or seeking more information or shared decision making. Remember the possible breast lump? What if you're sitting in the provider's office and she or he says, "the biopsy shows that lump is a cancer"—what would you hypothesize occurs at that moment in the patient's consciousness? Would it be surprising to learn that for many people the word *cancer* has terrifying connotations (relational meaning, e.g., that's what killed grandma, or I won't see my son get married) in addition to the denotative (dictionary) realities that overwhelm the brain's ability to process incoming information?

In interpersonal communication, verbalized messages generally have two distinct types of meaning—denotative and connotative. The denotative meaning is literally the dictionary definition, cancer is a disease in which cells divide abnormally and can destroy other cells and/or organs. However, the connotative meaning of a message is much more personal, abstract, and/or subjective. So to one person cancer might have a connotative meaning of death, that's what killed Aunt Helen, or long-term sickness from the chemotherapy. The connotative meaning often has little to do with the denotative meaning—it is much more of an emotional response based on a person's knowledge, experiences, hearsay, or myth. Thus, a provider may tell a patient that his or her breast tumor is a stage-zero carcinoma, noninvasive—compared to more advanced stages, this would be the best possible news for a patient. However, if the patient's connotative interpretation of the message is terminal cancer, it is highly unlikely that the patient will hear little if any of the information the provider attempts to communicate about the disease, treatment plans, or prognosis. In this context, the connotative meaning and the patient's emotional response have created so much noise in the interaction that she or he will not be able to process effectively the rest of the provider's information.

Reflection 3.6. If you are delivering potentially emotionally charged news to a patient and/or family member, how might you try to overcome that person's connotative response and obstructive noise in the interaction?

_____

_____

_____

_____

_____

Once we recognize how problematic noise can be to effective interpersonal communication—especially from unrecognized connotative miscommunication—we can begin to find ways to help avoid or deal with the issue. For example, if you have to deliver news to a patient that you think could trigger a negative emotional response, you can either try to verbalize the message in a way that addresses the potential connotative meaning and minimize or eliminate it. Another way to help assure that the patient gets the information she or he needs in spite of the likely noise from the connotative meaning of the message is to ask the patient to bring a relative with him or her to the interaction. The patient's advocate is generally less emotionally impacted because it is not directly affecting him or her, and therefore can listen more effectively, take notes, ask questions, and share the information with the patient at a later time in a different, less emotional setting. Also, it is often very helpful to have a handout that is language specific (English, Spanish, etc.) and written at an appropriate patient reading level that can be taken home and easily understood by the patient and his or her family. The importance of recognizing the potential negative impact of noise and connotative meanings on interactions will help you assess your patient/family member and determine the most effective way to communicate health information to help enhance the patient's assimilation and decision making.

Listening

Before we move to our discussion of nonverbal competencies, it is very important that we highlight the critical role listening plays in effective interpersonal communication, but also in interpersonal relationships. Listening is different from hearing. Hearing is anatomical and physiological—if you have ears and they are working normally—you can hear. However, listening requires attention and focus on the other communicator and the message. We've already discussed how emotional noise can interfere with patients' abilities to listen. But too often providers do not listen as effectively as they could. Some providers are so concerned with their needs to gather specific information and intrapersonally complete an algorithm based on the patient's complaints that they do not listen to all that the patient/family member is trying to communicate. In addition, with the use of computers in health care contexts, providers are frequently so preoccupied with completing the electronic document that their focus is on the computer instead of listening to the patient. And, as briefly mentioned earlier, like patients, providers can have extra conversation issues impact their listening. Problems with family, friends, finances, even other patients who are not doing well, all can create noise that can interfere with a provider's active listening. Finally, some providers may believe that the data they need to gather is more critical than the information the patient wants to share—in those cases the provider may minimize his or her listening and focus only on the responses that meet the provider's information-seeking needs.

All of these issues are potential obstructions to patient and provider listening and consequently effective interpersonal communication. Armed with this information, providers need to not only understand the importance of effective listening, but also to assure that they are doing all they can to enhance active listening. Some ways to improve your listening include:

- Making the patient's message your key focus
- Trying not to make your information needs more important than the patient's
- Waiting to type/write/focus on your computer or paper until the patient has finished speaking

- Using eye contact to demonstrate your listening
- Providing feedback (restating what you heard or asking questions, even nodding or shaking your head) to demonstrate listening and/or understanding/confusion

The use of feedback is an important tool to assure that you have assimilated what was communicated correctly, but also to reinforce for the patient/family member that you were listening and want to clarify. Feedback can also be used to check that the patient understood what you told him or her. For example, you can ask the patient to restate what you just communicated. Try to avoid simply asking whether she or he has any questions—too often patients/family members didn't understand what you said, or were unable to process the information because of noise, and they do not know what to ask, or want you to know that they didn't assimilate what you communicated. As you can tell, the importance of verbally sharing easily understood symbols, recognizing the importance of denotative versus connotative meanings in interactions, and the critical nature of listening are all necessary for competent verbal communicators. However, as valuable as effective verbal communication is to information exchanges, interpersonal communication, and interpersonal relationships—in the U.S. culture, nonverbal competencies are even more critical.

Nonverbal Communication

In American culture, nonverbal communication is extremely important to effective information exchange, interpersonal communication, and relationships. Nonverbal codes are used to express meaning, manage information flow, and contribute to or detract from verbal messages. As you know, we use nonverbal symbols to help receivers recognize whether we like or dislike something (e.g., smile, frown, thumbs-up), agree or disagree (e.g., head movement vertically versus horizontally), or are interested or disinterested in conversation (e.g., eye contact or body position/movements). Nonverbal behaviors also are used to illustrate power and status in this culture. For example, if you have a corner office at work or you are in a cubicle, your status in the organization is immediately recognized by your peers. In health care we use white coats, scrub clothes, and nametags to help patients and colleagues identify us as members of the provider culture and our printed credentials, MD, DO (doctor of osteopathy), RN, physician assistant (PA), advanced practice registered nurse (APRN), physical therapist (PT), to provide nonverbal information about our organizational status.

In terms of combined verbal and nonverbal messages together, interactants frequently use nonverbal codes to evaluate verbal messages. For example, if you are shaking your head from side to side, while you tell someone there is nothing to worry about—the other person is likely going to trust your nonverbal message more than your verbal statement and be concerned. So nonverbals can be used to reinforce verbal messages, contradict them, or highlight certain aspects of them. For example if you say "fire," others may think it is not a major problem. But if you say "fire!" and your voice rises both in pitch and volume, people are much more likely to not only perceive a problem, but respond immediately. The verbal symbol did not change, but the nonverbal cues, raising your voice and pitch, alerted listeners that this is not a typical use of the word *fire*. Be aware, however, that others can use your nonverbals in an interaction to also assess your credibility and interest. How would you feel if a health care provider, during an exam or discussion with a patient, goes to a closed exam room door and puts her or his hand on the knob while asking, "any questions"? In this culture, is there any reason to believe that this provider really wants questions? In fact, most patients would likely assume just the opposite—the nonverbal cue, hand on doorknob, is what the provider intends to communicate—I am leaving; not the verbal message: seeking more conversation. As you can see, our nonverbal behaviors in this culture are extremely important to the effectiveness of an information exchange. But, before we discuss nonverbals in more detail, there are two things that we absolutely need to be clear about:

1. Communication is about the receiver of the message, so it is not about what the sender of the message intends, it is about what the receiver understands. We can assume that in the previous example the provider did not intend to communicate that she or he was ready to close the conversation with no further dialogue, but, based on his or her nonverbal behavior, that is what the receiver (patient) perceived.

2. Everything we do communicates to others. Therefore, if you show up 5 minutes late for your first day of clinicals—whether you intended to or not—you have likely communicated to your superiors (and maybe even your peers) that you did not think it was worth your effort to get to the hospital/office on time.

The importance of these two realities is that a health care provider needs to be constantly aware of patients' and peers' perceptions of his or her message (verbal and nonverbal) and pay close attention to what is being communicated and how he or she intended the message to be interpreted.

Reflection 3.7. You are discussing a spinal tap procedure with a patient and she asks, "Does it hurt?" You respond, "Not really," but your eyes are looking away from the patient and you bite your lower lip as you finish speaking. What would you hypothesize a patient in this culture would perceive the answer to her question to be and why?

_____

_____

_____

_____

_____

In order to better understand nonverbal behaviors, it will be helpful to discuss them in the categories in which they are commonly used:

- Proxemics—related to the distance between interactants in a conversation
- Haptics—how touch is used in nonverbal communication
- Kinesics—the use of our bodies to communicate
- Artifacts—accessories that contribute to the information exchanged in an interaction
- Vocalics—the use of voice characteristics to alter message delivery
- Chronemics—the impact of time on message exchanges

While entire books are dedicated to the discussion of these important nonverbal behaviors, we need to explore in some detail how each of these impact interpersonal communication and, therefore, interpersonal relationship development, maintenance, and/or dissolution.

Proxemics

Proxemics is an important nonverbal cue for health care providers to understand. In American cultural research, Hall (1959) has shown that we have communication expectations based on very specific distances between interactants. Think about your own conversations and try to recall how far apart you stand/sit from a friend/lover/colleague/professional when you are engaged in an interpersonal conversation. Generally, in this culture, we expect to have about 4 to 12 feet between ourselves and another person in a social situation: restaurant, classroom, retail setting, and so forth. However, if we are talking with friends we are likely to be significantly closer, usually between 2 and 4 feet. Consequently, only our most intimate friends and lovers are generally expected in our private space, between 0 and 18 inches.

Research Exercise 3a. You are a social scientist and you want to study proxemics. Go to a retail setting, not a bar or club. Find a stranger of the same sex (very important—do not attempt this with a stranger of the opposite sex) and start a conversation. As you two are talking, *slowly* inch closer to the other person (very slowly). How close were you able to get? What happened? How did this research project make you feel and why?

_____

_____

_____

_____

_____

Reflection 3.8. As a health care provider, why would proxemics be important for you to understand? Have you thought about proximity in visits you have made to your own health care provider, or when you went to the emergency department (ED) or to a new provider? If so, what were your concerns?

_____

_____

_____

_____

_____

Proxemics, as you may have concluded, are extremely important nonverbal behaviors for health care providers to understand and utilize in interactions with patients. Think about your role in health care and how much of what you do involves "invading" a patient's personal space. From taking vital signs (pulse, temperature, and blood pressure), to auscultating the chest, and exercising joints, almost everything health care providers do involves behaviors that are unacceptable in any other context. Supposing you were on a bus and you approached a stranger and suddenly grabbed his or her wrist and began feeling for a pulse. Or you started doing range-of-motion exercises with his or her knee—do you think that person would respond positively to these nonverbal behaviors? In all likelihood, the person would either scream and push you away, or try to punch you for invading his or her space. Clearly, these actions in the context of a bus, that are done constantly in a health care setting, are made even more unacceptable because they include the use of haptics (touch), which, combined with inappropriate proxemics, compound the miscommunication and misperception of your actions. The question you need to ask yourself is: Do patients give up the right to expect input into this infringement on their personal space in a health care setting versus all other U.S. contexts (except prison)? This book is intended to help you assess the role of communication in such situations, especially in a health care context.

Now, it should be understood that if we are discussing a life or death emergency situation, then the provider should do whatever is needed to aid the patient. However, in the overwhelming majority of health delivery scenarios, providers all too often assume that their needs (to gather data) supersede the patients' perceptions of personal space and who can enter that domain without approval. In these instances, how much time would it take to acknowledge the patient's right to his or her space and ask permission to enter it? For example, a simple query like, "Is it alright with you if I pull my chair up closer so I can examine you?" This one-sentence verbal message does much more than just communicate your recognition of the patient's space. Such a question informs the patient that she or he has power in this interaction and that the two of you are collaborating in the process. When a provider invades a patient's space without acknowledging the patient's right to control his or her environment, the provider has nonverbally demonstrated his or her power as well as the patient's loss of autonomy and decision making. This single act contributes to a patient's assumption that the provider is taking an authoritarian role in the interaction and consequently is likely to be more paternalistic and declarative in his or her analysis, diagnosis, and treatment plan than informative, collaborative, and encouraging. Once a provider understands the importance of proxemics in this culture, she or he can make empowered decisions about how she or he wants, or does not want, to acknowledge the patient's personal space and the provider's need to access it. However, as noted earlier, proxemics is just one aspect of nonverbal behaviors—even more critical perhaps to patient–provider relationships and communication is the role of haptics.

Haptics

In the United States, touch (haptics) is generally reserved for close friends, family, and lovers. In fact, there are laws governing a person's right to control who touches him or her socially and professionally. If you recall our example of the aforementioned bus rider who is suddenly touched without his or her permission, you likely had an almost primal response to the thought of a stranger touching you without your permission. And yet, every day in this country health care providers do exactly that to patients. Think of the last time you took someone's blood pressure or went to draw blood—consider especially this latter behavior—you are going to cause someone pain and yet, if you are like the majority of providers in this county, you didn't ask to touch the person before you twisted a tourniquet around his or her arm tight enough to constrict the circulation and then inserted a needle into his or her vein (perhaps even without a warning that you were going to do that as well). Now, you can argue that a patient comes to see you for this very nonverbal behavior (to get his or her blood drawn), but does that mean she or he knowingly abdicated the right to say what happens to her or his body? If you recall the earlier discussion of all behaviors communicating—whether intended or not—what would you think a patient might perceive the message to be when a provider grabs his or her arm and performs a venipuncture without asking the patient's permission to invade his or her space and touch the arm? It seems fairly clear that such a behavior would again communicate that a provider thinks his or her actions are more important than the patient's autonomy. Once again, you as a provider have to make decisions about how you want to be perceived by patients, but if your actions (not seeking permission to touch) are so different from all other areas of American culture (except prison)—does it not seem wise to take a minute to explain to the patient that you need to draw blood, for example, and you would like his or her permission to touch the arm?

From a patient's perspective, think about how important it is to have a health care professional acknowledge the right to control what happens to the patient's body. Nonverbally it communicates the provider's desire to collaborate, not dictate, to a patient about his or her health care. It is so important to understand how each communication behavior (verbal and nonverbal) can be cumulative in terms of how a patient perceives a provider's empathy, compassion, and willingness to share power. As you may have noted, proxemics and haptics are two very important nonverbal behaviors in provider–patient communication, but there are several more, especially kinesics.

Reflection 3.9. How would you feel if you were in a classroom or continuing-education conference and the professor/presenter came over to you and grabbed your hand and started helping you write notes? Were you not in that environment to learn? So how is that use of haptics different or similar to the previous blood-drawing example?

_____

_____

_____

_____

_____

Kinesics

Although the term *kinesics* may not be familiar to you, the nonverbal communication behaviors it refers to will be. Some of the common actions included in kinesics include:

- Body movements
  - Gestures
  - Gaze
  - Facial expressions
  - Arms crossed on chest
  - Leaning back in a chair
  - Sitting with legs spread out

Research Exercise 3b. When you are in a meeting or in a classroom, put on your social scientist "hat" and observe how the speaker uses his or her kinesics to communicate with the audience. How do body movements and artifacts impact your perception of the speaker, the message, and the speaker's credibility (be as specific and detailed as possible)?

_____

_____

_____

_____

_____

Body Movements

Body movements refer to a person's posture and gait. In this culture, we use body movements as one way to determine a communicator's status, power, and interest. As mentioned previously, some people may not be consciously aware of these nonverbal behaviors, but their actions are nonetheless observed and assessed by others. Therefore, if you are in a meeting and you are sitting in a "closed" position (arms folded against your chest, legs crossed, pushed away from the table/desk), those body movements will likely be perceived as someone who is withdrawn or has little interest in what is being discussed. In contrast, if you are in a meeting and are leaning forward, with your arms and legs uncrossed, this "open" posture communicates your interest in the speaker and the topic and your attention to the material being presented. Similarly, if you are walking down the hall and moving slowly, your supervisor may perceive that you are bored or disinterested. How you move communicates to others and the more you understand that, the easier it will be for you to make decisions about how you want your body movements and gait to be perceived by others.

Another form of body movement that is highly assessed and perceived as a key nonverbal cue in this culture is the handshake. Americans believe that a firm handshake is an expected nonverbal form of greeting, especially between two interpersonal communicators. In general, a handshake is an anticipated communication when meeting someone, either for the first time in a professional context or as a traditional greeting in many interactions with friends, colleagues, clients, or customers. It is in fact one person offering another person the right to touch him or her (haptics). However, this aspect of kinesics is not just evaluated on whether it is communicated (an offer of a handshake or not), but equally for how strongly or weakly a person grips the other communicator if a handshake occurs. A weak handshake in this culture is often perceived as either a sign of disinterest, weakness, or diminished self-confidence.

Based on these expectations, you can not only observe how others use body movements in their interactions with you, but also be aware of how you use these forms of kinesics in your nonverbal communication. For health care professionals, kinesics is especially important as you need to observe your patients' body movements as part of your physical examination. You will want to determine, for example, whether a patient has a facial droop, or a limp, a weak grip, or an asymmetrical palpebral fissure (distance between eye lids). Although these kinesics may be signs of an illness or injury, they are also nonverbal behaviors that are communicating information about the patient. Therefore, you can use those same powers of health care observation to analyze kinesics (yours and others) during interpersonal interactions and evaluate what the body movements are communicating about the sender and his or her or your nonverbal messages. In this culture, another type of body movement that is perceived as having more credibility than others in the assessment of communication is one's gaze.

Gaze

In American culture, we highly value a person's gaze. This form of kinesics is generally theorized to communicate a person's honesty and/or credibility based on whether that person is willing to make eye contact during an interpersonal interaction. Consider for a moment a male patient whom you are interviewing and he is complaining of dysuria (painful urination). To learn more about his problem, you ask him whether he previously had a sexually transmitted disease (STD). As he starts to respond, you notice that his eyes are not looking at you, but instead, he is looking down at the floor, as he states, "Of course not!" This is an example of contradictory verbal and nonverbal cues. The patient has verbally denied any prior STD history, but his nonverbal kinesics (gaze), have suggested that he may not be telling the truth. Again, in this culture, we expect nonverbal behaviors to "complement" our verbal cues. Therefore, we expect people to look us in the eye when responding to questions—especially sensitive questions like the one in this scenario. When a person in a professional or personal setting does not use his or her gaze as expected in this culture that individual's communication is generally perceived negatively regardless of his or her verbal behaviors. Although body movements and gaze often work together to reinforce nonverbal messages, they also can be cumulative in connection with other forms of kinesics, for example, facial expressions.

Reflection 3.10. You have an interview for a job and go to greet the interviewer. Nonverbally, what are two of the most important kinesics you need to utilize to demonstrate your interest, sincerity, and recognition of cultural expectations for professional greetings?

_____

_____

_____

_____

_____

Facial Expressions

Although in American culture there is an added emphasis placed on the assessment of nonverbal cues based on a communicator's gaze, the importance of a communicator's facial expressions in transmitting his or her meaning is also very important to understand. Facial expressions are powerful nonverbal cues, especially in terms of communicating understanding, confusion, and emotions.

If you recall a recent conversation, professional or personal, you can likely remember how a colleague, supervisor/professor, friend, or lover responded during an interpersonal interaction. In this culture, we generally seek nonverbal feedback in a conversation by observing the other communicator for a smile or a frown, a grimace, or raised eyebrows, and so forth. Similarly, we often assess a person's facial expression to deduce whether she or he is happy, sad, angry, fearful, surprised, or disgusted. As an interpersonal communicator and a health care professional, you will want to utilize these various forms of nonverbal behaviors to help you better understand your patients' and peers' communication, but also to recognize how your own use of kinesics (facial expressions) are being analyzed by others. As mentioned previously, communicators use nonverbal cues to demonstrate and to analyze the assimilation of information, impact of the message on others, and/or the disconnect between a speaker's verbal and nonverbal cues. A patient who has a pensive look on his or her face (wrinkled forehead, pursed lips, raised brows) may be trying to "unpack" the meaning of what was just heard. Or she or he may be confused about what was stated. In either case, a thoughtful interpersonal communicator might ignore the patient's verbal ascent of understanding and use kinesics to determine that more clarity and content are needed to better assure effective assimilation of the message. Similar to body movements and gaze, facial expressions offer communicators both an opportunity to share information nonverbally, but also provide a feedback mechanism to help assess a person's recognition and understanding of the message. However, not all nonverbal behaviors are feedback mechanisms. Specifically, artifacts are more (consciously and/or subconsciously) communicator-centric forms of nonverbal communication.

Artifacts

Artifacts refer to a wide array of nonverbal cues, including body types, clothing, jewelry, and body adornments (tattoos, piercings, and so forth). By their very nature, artifacts tend to be a person's communication about himself or herself to others (specific or in general). For example, a 20-year-old co-ed wearing bright-pink sweat pants with the word "Party" in big white letters across her butt probably did not consider how that would be perceived by a 60-year-old male professor walking up the stairs directly behind her. It is unlikely that this woman intended, when she got dressed that day, to either invite the professor to "party" or to make him aware of her extracurricular proclivities. And yet, that is exactly what her artifacts have communicated. Similarly, what about an emergency department (ED) provider who walks around in scrub clothes with his tattoos (neck and arms) and piercings (eyebrows, ears, and tongue) visible—do you think patients or even peers might perceive him as less credible a professional because of his body art? And what about the potential risk of hepatitis C from tattoos and piercings—might patients be somewhat concerned for their health? Although such an infection risk from tattoo needles, and so forth may be extremely low, it is a possibility and so is the perception of provider–patient transmission—which could be communicated nonverbally by the provider's artifacts.

Reflection 3.11. Why is it that health care organizations have certain dress codes regarding white coats, scrub clothes, uniforms, jewelry, and so forth? What is the organization trying to nonverbally communicate to its members and to its patients and their family members?

_____

_____

_____

_____

_____

Unlike other forms of kinesics, artifacts are more subjective. For example, in this culture we have research that shows how people generally perceive limp handshakes, down-turned gazes, and frowns versus smiles, but artifacts are much more individualized. If a person is a fan of tattoos or piercings, then another person's body art might very well be perceived as a positive nonverbal behavior. However, to a different person, who is not a fan of body art, tattoos, and piercings, they could be viewed as negative nonverbal messages. Therefore, health care professionals need to understand both what they are communicating with their artifacts and how they are assessing their patients' and peers' artifacts. It is important to not stereotype and certainly it would be a huge communication mistake to evaluate everyone who is obese as uncaring about his or her health. Or to categorize everyone who is thin as anorexic or bulimic. However, at the same time, it is important for providers to understand how patients, peers, family members, and/or organization administrators might perceive the providers' artifacts. How do you think a 200-pound male patient might assess the verbal versus nonverbal (body type) artifact communication from a female provider who weighs 300 pounds and tells the patient that he needs to lose weight to stay healthy? As stated previously, it is impossible not to communicate (whether intended or not), so in order to be a skilled, thoughtful, interpersonal communicator—you need to understand how your nonverbal cues, including your artifacts, are impacting others' perceptions and determine whether that is the message you want to be sending. However, not all nonverbal behaviors are silent, in fact, vocalics are an auditory form of nonverbal communication.

Vocalics

It may seem odd that there are sounds that are classified as nonverbal communication; however, it really makes sense when you consider _how_ we say things is sometimes more communicative than the verbal symbols we use. For example, "I need some help in here," may be a simple request for some assistance by one provider to another, but the same symbols—when screamed at the highest volume a person can reach—communicate an emergent level of need. The various nonverbal characteristics (e.g., volume, pitch, and inflection) of our voices allow us to alter the way in which our verbal messages are perceived. In addition, communicators can use laughing, crying, and whining as nonverbal behaviors to transmit both physical (tears) and/or emotional feelings. Health care providers need to be aware of how vocalics can be used to impact communication exchanges. Think about how your response to paralinguistic cues (screaming, crying, whining, laughing, and so forth) might impact your communication and/or your feedback to a sender's message. Another unique form of nonverbal communication is related to the use of time—chronemics.

Reflection 3.12. How do you respond when you are in a conversation with a person who is crying? What if that person is a patient, would you respond differently? If so, how and why is the same nonverbal cue different?

_____

_____

_____

_____

_____

Chronemics

In America, we have some very specific views on how we use time. For example, if you are expected to be at work or in class at 8:30 a.m., arriving at 8:45 a.m. is generally viewed negatively and consequently may impact your pay, promotion, grade, and so forth. In health care, time can be a critical factor, for example, defibrillation that is delayed a few minutes could be the difference between life and death. Medication is usually most effective when provided on a set schedule and, similarly, the amount of radiation exposure is time dependent. However, although these are obvious impacts of time on treatment outcomes in health care delivery, _chronemics_ refers to the use of time as a form of nonverbal communication.

One of the most frequent patient complaints in providers' offices and hospital settings is related to chronemics. Patients and family members often perceive delayed appointments/visits with providers as nonverbal communication of the power and status differences in provider–patient interactions. Think about meetings or classes you attend, they generally do not begin until the leader/supervisor/professor arrives. Clearly, if she or he is leading the discussion or scheduled the gathering, then the perception is that nothing can take place until the person in charge arrives. Consequently, the audience in this case is aware of the leader's/professor's power and control over when things will begin and end. As a person who does not control the timing of these events, how do you feel when you arrive on time, but the featured speaker/ leader does not? Or you get summoned to your supervisor's/professor's office and when you arrive, you are asked to sit and wait until she or he is ready to see you—what do those nonverbal cues communicate to you (come to the office, wait till I am ready)? If you are like most Americans, and have been summoned and told to wait until the other communicator is ready, you perceive these behaviors as an illustration of that person's power and status.

From a nonverbal perspective, being a patient is even more difficult and frustrating. First, the patient is the person who is paying (insurance, copay, Medicare, etc.) for a service—which has its own set of expectations in this culture—but is unlike other contexts (e.g., a retail store where a sales person does not arrive in a timely manner to assist you). Second, the patient may be in pain, or anxious about the reason for the visit. Third, the patient is probably partially naked as she or he waits for the provider. Consequently, it is very difficult in such a scenario for a patient to walk out of an ED or a provider's office because the patient is unhappy with the wait or being treated less than an equal. Therefore, through the use of chronemics, the provider has reinforced his or her power and/or status vis-à-vis the nonverbal communication that her or his time is more valuable than the patient's time. If you were in an interpersonal relationship (friend, lover, colleague) and the other person used chronemics to control the start and close of conversations, would you want to maintain or end that relationship?

As we have been discussing throughout this chapter, nonverbal communication is a powerful tool for enhancing or diminishing interpersonal relationships. A provider who schedules a patient visit every 10 minutes but knows that he or she will keep patients waiting is clearly more provider-centric than patient focused and communicates that reality to patients and staff through his or her use of chronemics. Clearly, verbal and nonverbal communications are critically important for effective patient–provider interactions and relationship development and maintenance. But interpersonal communication also relies on communicators understanding their roles, selves, and competencies.

Research Exercise 3c. Ask three people (a parent/grandparent, a peer, and a health care provider) the same question: "Why do doctors so often make patients wait before they see them?" and analyze their answers. What did you learn from the various audience responses/perceptions?

_____

_____

_____

_____

_____

■ ROLE, SELF, AND GOAL COMPETENCIES

Part of being an effective interpersonal communicator as well as a successful health care professional is possessing communication competence as demonstrated through your understanding of role, self, and goal proficiencies. _Role_ *competence* refers to a person's ability to take on certain social roles (e.g., friend, parent, professional) and what the expected behaviors for each are, how to maintain them, and when it is okay to ignore those norms.

Think of your role as a health care provider, how does that shape your behavior—especially your interpersonal communication and relationship development? Do you use your role to highlight your status and power (verbally and nonverbally) or do you use your role to help you collaborate, empower, and educate patients? If you see your role as the person responsible for solving patient's problems, making decisions for them, and being in control—you will likely assume a much more authoritarian position in your interactions with patients and family members. In contrast, if you see your role as participative you will be much more likely to take on a collaborative focus in your communication with patients and families. Therefore, the way you perceive your role in health care is going to have a direct impact on how you communicate. Providers have been often criticized for being disease focused and consequently seeing their role as more problem solving than information- and power-sharing collaborators. Just because you are licensed/certified to be a health care provider your role competency is going to be determined by how you choose to communicate that position to others. However, in addition to your role impacting your interpersonal communication, so does your self-competence.

Self-competence is related to the self-image you choose to present to others. Based on your self-competence you can use interpersonal communication to determine how others perceive you. For example, in your health care provider role, you can decide that you want to be seen as an intellectual, authority figure who knows more than patients and therefore you can unilaterally make decisions for them and share only the information you think is needed. Or you may want to present yourself as a patient-focused partner in health care delivery who encourages a dialogue, information and power sharing, as well as collaborative decision making. However, equally important as role and self-competence is goal competence.

Goal competence is knowing how to attain your communication goals. This means you are able to utilize both your American English-language literacy and your audience analysis to communicate effectively with the intended interactant. Therefore, you must rely on your interpersonal communication and relationship development skills, as well as your self- and role competencies to become goal competent. As this chapter has pointed out, being an effective interpersonal communicator is much more than knowing about health care. Instead, to be successful when interacting with patients, family members, and peers it is critically important to not only assess their needs, literacy levels, and knowledge of the topic, but your own role and self-competence in order to attain your communication goals. However, in addition to assessing the other communicator from a content/capability focus, you also need to be able to determine how a person's gender may impact his or her communication behaviors.

◼ SEX VERSUS GENDER

In U.S. culture, we frequently confuse the terms *sex* and *gender*. However, from a social science and especially a communication perspective—these terms can be very different and yet critically important to effective interpersonal communication and relationship development. As Wood (2015) points out, "sex is a designation based on biology, whereas gender is socially constructed and expressed" (p. 19). This is truly important for health care providers. As you likely have seen, for nearly 100% of the population, sex can be determined based on the presence of a penis (male) or a vagina (female). For the very small minority of individuals who have unique genitalia, the older term *hermaphrodite* has been replaced with the current classification of *intersexed*. This text will not be exploring the social, psychological, and communication behaviors associated with being born intersexed. However, it is very important that health care providers recognize that just because an individual has a penis, he may or may not communicate using masculine-gendered behaviors. And the same is true for a female, her sex does not define her gender—like males, her behaviors do.

And because gender is socially constructed, it can evolve and change as a person matures, has new experiences, and is more aware of his or her own feelings. Gender identity is an individual's understanding of himself or herself. In our culture, we traditionally identify being masculine as strong, independent, aggressive, and unwilling to share many emotions, whereas being feminine is more about physical appearance, nurturing, showing emotions, and an interest in relationship development/maintenance. There are a number of theories regarding these gendered behaviors and how from infancy to adulthood we learn how to be masculine, feminine, or somewhere along that spectrum.

> **Reflection 3.13.** Think about your own gender identity. Do you perceive yourself as more masculine or feminine? What behaviors or feelings do you use to illustrate one gender over the other? Are there contexts in which you may need to behave the opposite of what you feel is the norm for you (more masculine if you see yourself as feminine, or vice versa)? If so, why? If not, why not?

Some of the theories of gender, include:

- Biological
- Psychodynamic

- Social learning
- Cognitive development

These theories provide us with a breadth of views on how gender is developed, constructed, and evolves. Let's examine the distinctions among them and how they can help you better understand your patients, peers, and others to be able to communicate more effectively with them.

Biological theory promotes the view that gender behaviors are the result of physiological processes (e.g., hormones, genetics). According to biological theory, hormones like testosterone and estrogen are responsible in part for gendered actions. So changes in testosterone levels, for example, could result in more or less aggression, nurturing, and so forth. But in addition, this theory also proposes that anatomy, specifically brain development, has a role in gender determination. As you may know, males tend to have better developed left lobes and therefore are often more linear, spatial, and abstract in their thinking. Females have increased right lobes, which control imagination and creativity among other cognitive functions. Clearly, there are some reasons to support biological theory, but it is also true that there are other theoretical possibilities for how gender behaviors are developed.

Psychodynamic theory centers around the importance of the mother–child relationship in the child's gender development. This theory proposes that female children are able to identify more closely anatomically with their mother and therefore tend to identify with their mother's gendered behaviors. Conversely, boys do not identify as closely with mom and therefore seek a father or other male figure as a guide. However, this theory also suggests that mothers realize the differences in gender and what is expected of males and encourage boys to behave differently than females. For example, boys are sent outside by their mother to play alone or with friends, whereas girls are encouraged to stay inside and help cook. But psychodynamic theory is not the only nonbiologic approach to gender development.

Social learning theory postulates that humans learn how to be masculine or feminine by watching others as children and then, using the feedback they receive for those behaviors to determine whether or not to adopt them. For example, a young boy might see his father watching a football game and enjoying it. Consequently, if he starts throwing a football or tackling his brother or friends and he gets positive feedback from his parents, friends, and siblings, according to this theory, he will likely see those behaviors as being appropriate for his gender. Conversely, if a girl sees a woman on TV fighting and she starts to fight with her sibling, she might get reprimanded by her parents, friends, and/or siblings for not being feminine and decide that those behaviors are incorrect for her gender. Although biological, psychodynamic, and social learning theories all suggest that outside forces are in large part responsible for the development of gendered behaviors, cognitive development theory is more person-centric.

Cognitive development theory suggests that children are not just responding to hormones and/or the directives or rewards of others, but actively developing their own gender identities. According to this theory, children listen and observe how others communicate with them and then pick which behaviors to continue in order to get the responses they desire (e.g., "a good little boy," or "a smart little girl"). According to this theory, children develop a sense of their gender very early, before they start kindergarten or first grade at the latest. However, regardless of which gender theory you support, the important aspect for those in health care is that gender shapes our lives, communication, and decision making and it cannot be deduced by merely observing a person's sex. Therefore, it is very important for you as a health care professional to understand differences in masculine- and feminine-gendered behaviors and not stereotype all males as masculine or all females as feminine.

■ MASCULINE- VERSUS FEMININE-GENDERED COMMUNICATION

Although it is crucial for providers to understand the differences between gender and sex, as well as the theories of gender development, it is equally if not more essential that health care professionals recognize the distinctions between feminine and masculine communication behaviors. By doing so, providers can assess how those actions might impact patient information exchange, collaboration, trust, and/or decision making. In America, feminine communication is typically used to nurture and develop relationships (familial, platonic, and/or romantic), whereas masculine communication refers to behaviors that generally support the speaker's independence, control, goals, and status. One of the key masculine behaviors that demonstrate control is how often masculine-gendered individuals interrupt others. Also, masculine speech is more often to the point and more forceful than feminine-gendered communication. Conversely, feminine-behaviors are more typically cultivating, collaborative, and encourage participation. Once health care providers begin to assess an individual's communication behaviors, not merely based on his or her sex, they can begin to better determine how to share information, power, and decision making.

By evaluating a patient's or peer's gender, vis-à-vis her or his communication, health care providers can determine the most effective communication style needed to meet the patient's expectations and desires. For example, if a provider is having a conversation with a feminine-gendered individual (female or male), the professional would want to understand the importance of building a relationship from the patient's perspective: having a provider who listens and offers feedback and is more interested in collaboration than an authoritative style. Similarly, if the provider determines that a patient is masculine gendered, regardless of his or her sex, then the professional would want to encourage more discussion, ask more questions, as well as enhance the patient's feeling of independence and control.

As we have been discussing, interpersonal communication is intended not just to build relationships, exchange information, and help interactants attain shared goals—it is also an opportunity to develop trust, promote credibility, and highlight similarities. The more your patients can feel that you are communicating interpersonally with them as individuals (based on their education, health literacy, age, and gender), the more likely it is that you can develop a trusting, collaborative relationship that will allow for the open exchange of information, power, control, and decision making.

It is important to recognize that one of the key aspects of developing and maintaining an interpersonal relationship is the use of self-disclosure. Communicators tend to use self-disclosure (of their most personal information) only with the most trusted people in their lives. Generally speaking, Americans self-disclose their most intimate life stories with a very few (one or two) extremely selective (platonically related, but more frequently romantically related) individuals. In fact, self-disclosure is one way of assessing how an interpersonal relationship is evolving. When one communicator chooses to self-disclose (e.g., I had an abortion or I was arrested, or I love you) in a burgeoning relationship—it is expected to help the relationship continue to grow. However, that expectation is dependent on the other interactant reciprocating with his or her own self-disclosure (building trust and helping ensure confidentiality). This is one of the tools we use in relationships to build reliance—sharing our most intimate feelings and/or experiences.

Reflection 3.14. Think of a relationship you have been in, either platonic or romantic. Can you recall when you or the other person made a self-disclosure and how it impacted the relationship (positively or negatively)? Was there a reciprocal self-disclosure? If so, did the presence or absence of a reciprocal response enhance the relationship or jeopardize it, and why?

_____

_____

_____

_____

_____

If self-disclosure is so key to developing and maintaining interpersonal relationships in the larger U.S. culture, then how does that impact your use of interpersonal communication in health care contexts? As should be somewhat obvious, health care providers do not just need a patient to self-disclose his or her most intimate experiences, they actually seek that information. Therefore, in a culture in which self-disclosure is limited to a communicator's closest friends and/or lovers, health care expects patients to communicate completely differently—telling providers (often strangers or near strangers), the most intimate details of a person's life (medical, sexual, psychological, family, etc.). No one in this culture, except health care professionals, routinely asks a person how many people she or he had sex with, if the patient has or had an STD or abortion, how much alcohol she or he consumes, or whether there is a present or past history of drug abuse or addiction by the patient or his or her family. But unlike every other interpersonal relationship in American culture, a unilateral self-disclosure by the patient is not only expected but professionally mandated. Therefore, think about how you might help maintain the relationship by explaining briefly the need for such private information, or assuring the patient that you will keep his or her disclosure confidential (keeping in mind that your records will be reviewed by the patient's insurance carrier, so there is only so much confidentiality possible). The point of this discussion is to remind you that health care occurs in a totally different context and requires much different interpersonal communication for patients than all other experiences in their lives (except perhaps jail).

Interpersonally, health care providers not only ask but expect patients to get naked, or nearly naked, allow themselves to be touched in areas usually restricted to a person's most intimate lovers, and self-disclose their most private experiences. However, at the same time the provider is trying to encourage the patient to develop/maintain a relationship with a communicator who is fully clothed, not touched by the patient (except perhaps for a handshake), and not reciprocating with her or his intimate personal data. Armed with these major deviations from expected interpersonal communication and relationship development in this culture, it should not be too surprising that there are not only health literacy issues that constrain provider–patient information exchanges and relationship development, but interpersonal communication expectations and experiences as well. As you work to become more effective interpersonal communicators and health care providers, try to remind yourselves of the importance of verbal and nonverbal cues, as well as gendered behaviors in not only assessing your patients' communication, but your own. In order to enhance patient outcomes and provide a context in which information is exchanged, provider–patient interactions are collaborative and informative and based on power equality and shared decision making, providers need to recognize their key role in assuring that messages are clear, complete, and effectively communicated based on the patient's health and language literacy, and assimilated appropriately. With such efforts, patients and providers have a much greater potential for attaining shared outcomes (e.g., wellness, and/or illness/injury treatment, goals).

Reflections (among the possible responses)

3.1. Thinking about a single interaction (with your provider, a colleague provider, or with a patient), how would you describe the communication exchange? Was it effective or problematic and why?

When you considered your prior interaction, if you looked at it as a patient, you likely had a completely different response than if you examined the conversation from a provider's perspective. That is why it is important to think about provider–patient communication from an interpersonal, not strictly diagnostic or treatment, perspective. The more you can attempt to find an equal power/

control viewpoint for your patient interactions the more the interpersonal communication becomes about exchanging information and accomplishing patient-centered goals. The problem with provider-focused communication is that the conversation is not about sharing, but about getting the data the provider needs so she or he can make a diagnosis, determine a treatment plan, and so forth and, therefore, collaborative and participative decision making is hardly possible.

3.2. Can you recall a situation in which you needed help from someone, or that person offered advice about something? Did/would your reactions to that offer change based on an interpersonal relationship with that person? If so, why? If not, why not?

Interpersonal communication research has shown that people are more likely to trust someone they have an interpersonal relationship with and therefore are more likely to carefully consider any recommendations or information from that person. Also, the more we like someone, the more we see that person as similar to ourselves and the more likely we are to share information and decision making with him or her. If a stranger spends 5 minutes with you and then tells you to take a pill and you will be better— are you not less likely to trust that recommendation than if you hear similar suggestions from a provider you have known for a longer period of time, who you like, who cares about you, and has your best interests in mind? If the stranger is seen as just another provider and not someone who cares about the uniqueness of the patient and his or her complaints, it is unlikely the patient is going to value highly, or even follow the provider-stranger's recommendation/advice. Using interpersonal communication (verbal and nonverbal) to develop and maintain a relationship has the most potential for accomplishing both your and the patient's shared health/wellness goals.

3.3. If you are in a relationship (platonic or romantic) and the other person self-discloses something very personal, what do you think that person expects in return? Why would that reality make it even harder for patients to self-disclose to providers?

In American culture, we expect the other person in a romantic or platonic relationship with us to reciprocate when we self-disclose. And yet, in health care contexts for a number of personal, psychological, and organizational reasons, providers are taught not to reciprocate, but instead make sure they get their patients to self-disclose information that no one else save maybe one or two other people even know. Once again, assume the role of patient, if a provider whom you do not know well, or who does not communicate any interest in forming an interpersonal relationship with you, asks you to disclose details of your sex life, alcohol and/or drug use, and will not be reciprocating, would you be as likely to share that information with him or her as you would with a provider you felt you had a trusting/caring relationship with? In most cases, having an emotional connection enhances trust and encourages information sharing—even when the provider cannot reciprocate.

3.4. Besides literacy, what do you think is another major obstacle in the health care context for effective interpersonal communication and information exchange?

There are many obstacles to effective interpersonal communication and information exchange in health care settings; among the most obvious are the patient's perceived loss of power and control. Patients often experience a diminished sense of autonomy based on a number of verbal and nonverbal factors in many health communication contexts. First and foremost is the issue of a clothed provider and a nearly naked patient. Second is the fact that many providers choose to stand over a patient (seated or reclining) clearly demonstrating the provider's power/control. Third, many providers use closed-ended questions to control the conversation—the provider determines what is important information and seeks to minimize any emotional or relational aspects not directly related to the provider's data-gathering needs. Fourth, providers frequently interrupt patients in order to control the conversation, time, and demonstrate nonverbally/verbally their power in the interaction. Finally, more often than not providers control both the openings (they almost always show up to the conversation *after* the patient has arrived) and closings—providers decide when their information-seeking/sharing needs are met and decide it is time to close the interaction (e.g., "any more questions?" with a hand on the door knob—mismatched verbal/nonverbal behaviors). Therefore, although health literacy is extremely important to effective provider–patient interactions, the impact of the provider's communication of power and control can be equally as obstructive to effective information-sharing and collaborative decision making.

3.5. Can you recall an exam or a lecture during which you had trouble concentrating because of something that had happened in your life? What was causing your distraction (a breakup with a lover, a death of a loved one, other unexpected joyous or sad news)?

Most of us have been in situations in which we had trouble concentrating on what was going on around us because of intrapersonal communication—usually unspoken dialogue with ourselves. Therefore, we can understand how difficult it is to listen and assimilate information when we are distracted by these emotional or physical interferences (noise). Consequently, as a health care provider it should not be surprising that many patients, even family members, have similar difficulties concentrating and understanding information presented along with a perceived or real life-threatening or life-changing diagnosis, prognosis, and/or treatment plan. If you are taking a test or listening to a lecture and you get distracted by some emotional or physical event in your life, it is problematic but far less serious than the reality for patients who are told they have a tumor, cancer, heart attack, and so forth. If you have difficulty concentrating because your significant other wants out of a relationship—imagine what it must be like for a patient who is just told she or he has a malignancy or his or her death is imminent? Health communication differs from all other forms of communication because of the emotional aspects of the context and content. Therefore, providers need to fully consider how to deliver "bad news" or potentially bad news to patients. Perhaps the provider will need to ask the patient to bring an advocate (spouse/family member/friend) to listen, take notes, and/or ask questions. Or the provider will decide to share the news, but request a second meeting the following day to assure the patient not only heard the message but also assimilated it correctly and has a chance to ask his or her questions and gather more information. One thing the provider should try to avoid is giving bad news and expecting the patient to make a carefully considered decision immediately thereafter. Unless the problem is a life or death situation, the provider would be wise to separate the information about the illness or injury from a detailed discussion about possible next steps and/or treatment options. The impact of "noise" in a communication channel, for example, the emotional fears attached to hearing certain words: *tumor, cancer, malignancy, heart attack, stroke,* and so forth—should suggest to providers the need to reassess how much information to provide at one time, the need for a patient advocate, the value of a repeat visit and further information sharing, and/or the value of literacy/language-appropriate handouts. The obfuscation created by potentially life-altering diagnoses, prognoses, and treatment options should suggest to providers the need to find alternative ways to communicate with patients and/or family members/advocates. Just being correct in a diagnosis should not be sufficient for a provider—the patient needs to be able to understand what has been determined, assimilate the facts and the options, and make an informed decision. However, without adequate time and appropriate contexts, patients cannot be expected to quickly overcome their initial reactions/fears/uncertainties and address important decision-making options while they are still unable to fully process information and respond appropriately to it.

3.6. If you are delivering potentially emotionally charged news to a patient and/or family member, how might you try to overcome that person's connotative response and obstructive noise in the interaction?

In such a scenario, a health care provider would be wise to recognize the risk of emotional noise and/or fear in the conversation and do all she or he can to minimize that possibility. As mentioned earlier, you could encourage the patient to bring an advocate (spouse, life partner, friend, etc.) to listen, take notes, and discuss with the patient what had been discussed with the provider at a later time in a different setting. And you might ask yourself whether you are doing all you can to encourage assimilation of information. For example, did you schedule the time to talk about the emotionally charged news when you have time to sit and answer all the patient's/family's questions and provide feedback to determine what the patient/family member heard, understood, and/or had questions about? Are you attentive to your language choices and use verbal messages that are both literacy and language appropriate? Do you need a professional translator? Be sure to pay close attention to your nonverbal behaviors so you are communicating more collaboratively and less authoritatively/paternalistically—sit, maintain eye contact, encourage questions, make sure your nonverbal behaviors are complementary, not contradictory, communicate your empathic listening by allowing the patient/family member to fully express his or her feelings, concerns, and questions. Provide further information in print for later reading, again based on the educational, language, and literacy levels of the patient/family. Offer to answer questions at a later time by phone or in person. Be careful not to provide unrealistic hope or expectations, but focus on quality-of-life issues and empowering the patient to aid him or her in making informed decisions.

3.7. You are discussing a spinal tap procedure with a patient and she asks, "Does it hurt?" You respond, "Not really," but your eyes are looking away from the patient and you bite your lower lip as you finish speaking. What would you hypothesize a patient in this culture would perceive the answer to her question to be and why?

As discussed earlier, nonverbal communication/behavior in U.S. culture is perceived as more accurate than verbal messages. Therefore, a provider who says one thing, but nonverbally contradicts the statement is most likely communicating the opposite of what she or he said. Consequently, providers need to be keenly aware of the importance of complementing their verbal messages with appropriate nonverbal cues. In the context described in this question it is likely that the provider did not want to scare the patient by honestly communicating the reality: "There will be some pain, discomfort, and/or pressure, but I will inject some medicine under your skin to make the pain less and I will tell you everything I am doing, before I do it." By communicating what you will be doing and what should be expected, both verbally and nonverbally, not only can the patient increase his or her trust in you, but he or she will be adequately informed of what is about to happen. Providers must resist the impulse to hide facts from patients, verbally or nonverbally, and instead find a way to empower the patient with information that can be understood, assimilated, and assessed. You may not be able to eliminate all pain in health care procedures and diagnostic tests, but you can make sure your patient is properly informed and prepared without having to interpret conflicting verbal and nonverbal messages.

3.8. As a health care provider, why would proxemics be important for you to understand? Have you thought about proximity in visits you have made to your own health care provider, or when you went to the emergency department (ED) or to a new provider? If so, what were your concerns?

Proxemics or the space between communicators is very important to provider–patient communication and relationship development. As discussed earlier, providers—in order to do their work—need to use haptics and proxemics to assess patients' vital signs, breath and heart sounds, abdomen, skin, and so forth. However, providers can either nonverbally demonstrate their power and control by touching the patient and altering the expected distances between communicators without asking the patient's permission, or providers can ask to infringe on the patient's personal space in order to do their exams. Taking a few seconds to illustrate providers' recognition of patients' proxemics and their expectations by asking permission to touch prior to doing so, is one small step in affording patients a bit of social/cultural normalcy and control.

3.9. How would you feel if you were in a classroom or continuing-education conference and the professor/presenter came over to you and grabbed your hand and started helping you write notes? Were you not in that environment to learn? So how is that use of haptics different or similar to the previous blood-drawing example?

Not unlike Reflection 3.8, this example seeks to help health care providers understand how touching someone, even if they have chosen to put themselves in the context, can be perceived and treated by the person in charge as a nonverbal permission to touch without asking. However, the act of acknowledging the patients' rights to control who touches their bodies, just as they do in all other aspects of their lives, demonstrate providers' recognition of power- and control-sharing in the provider–patient interaction.

3.10. You have an interview for a job and go to greet the interviewer. Nonverbally, what are two of the most important kinesics you need to utilize to demonstrate your interest, sincerity, and recognition of cultural expectations for professional greetings?

Two of the most important kinesics for greeting a stranger, or anyone for that matter, would be eye contact and a smile. Clearly, an applicant for a job wants to demonstrate his or her interest in the position, friendly/positive attitude, and honesty vis-à-vis his or her nonverbal behaviors. In U.S. culture, eye contact is perceived as critical to a communicator's assessment of the other person's interest, honesty, and credibility. A person's smile, or lack thereof, is assumed to reflect the individual's attitude and enthusiasm. Therefore, if these kinesic behaviors are recognized as being so vital to communicating these nonverbal messages in other aspects of a provider's life, why would she or he not want to use them also in his or her interactions with patients—both strangers and those who are well known? Try to find a way to use normative communication behaviors of the larger American culture in your microlevel interactions with patients—regardless of the context (ED, office, hospital, etc.)—and patients will likely appreciate your efforts to normalize the interaction.

3.11. Why is it that health care organizations have certain dress codes regarding white coats, scrub clothes, uniforms, jewelry, and so forth? What is the organization trying to nonverbally communicate to its members and to its patients and their family members?

Health care organizations are trying to establish the values, beliefs, and goals for their members, customers, and vendors, as well as meet regulatory requirements. Consequently, many institutions want to assure that their employees' artifacts: clothes, hair, jewelry, body art, and so forth meet the organization's, regulators', and patients' expectations. The need to find nonverbal ways to build credibility with customers is also a concern. Having standardized artifacts helps to both brand the organization and minimize employees' and customers'/patients' distractions. Finally, the more employees/providers appear professional, the more likely the perception that they are knowledgeable, well trained, and dedicated to the organization's values and goals.

3.12. How do you respond when you are in a conversation with a person who is crying? What if that person is a patient, would you respond differently? If so, how and why is the same nonverbal cue different?

One of the things a health care provider, or anyone for that matter, can do when a person is crying is acknowledge the person's sadness and encourage him or her to talk about what is causing the feelings. Or, in the case of a patient or a patient's family member, the provider knows why the person is crying—the provider can acknowledge the cause (fear, sorrow, pain, loss, etc.). Empathic listening allows providers to communicate their understanding of the patient's situation and feelings. Many times when someone is crying she or he just wants to be able to talk about his or her concerns with someone. The patient does not necessarily expect the other person to fix the problem/situation, but just to allow him or her to verbalize what is causing the feelings and tears. Clearly, if the patient is crying because of pain or a misunderstanding, a provider who listens can provide relief (medication and/or communication/education); however, providers need to be willing to ask questions when they are faced with a crying patient and/or family member and not ignore or avoid him or her. Building an interpersonal relationship in provider–patient interactions is no different from the nonverbal and verbal interpersonal communication required among friends, family, and/or lovers. Providers need to listen and offer patients an opportunity to discuss their situations/problems/concerns.

3.13. Think about your own gender identity. Do you perceive yourself as more masculine or feminine? What behaviors or feelings do you use to illustrate one gender over the other? Are there contexts in which you may need to behave the opposite of what you feel is the norm for you (more masculine if you see yourself as feminine, or vice versa)? If so, why? If not, why not?

In terms of how you think of your gender, do you see yourself as more competitive or collaborative? Are you more independent or participative? Do you strive to be more aggressive or nurturing? These are just some of the behaviors that distinguish masculine- from feminine-gendered individuals. However, as discussed earlier, you likely use a mixture of gendered behaviors and can position yourself somewhere along the gendered communication spectrum from über masculine to über feminine. Nonetheless, there are contexts when more masculine-gendered behaviors (regardless of a person's sex) may be the most appropriate—for example, in a crisis. If there is a fire and you need everyone to evacuate, you likely will want a more masculine-gendered communication style to assure that whoever is in the dwelling understands that they need to leave immediately and aggressively help anyone who may have difficulty getting out. Or if you are trying to encourage maximum participation in a team that you are leading, you may want to use a more feminine-gendered approach (regardless of your sex) and encourage collaboration and participation instead of using an authoritarian/paternalistic style. These same considerations can be applied to provider–patient and provider–provider interactions. There may be certain contexts in which it is important for you to assume a more masculine-gendered communication style, but in general, a more feminine approach allows for more collaboration, nurturing of the provider–patient relationship, and mutual participation in information sharing and decision making.

3.14. *Think of a relationship you have been in, either platonic or romantic. Can you recall when you or the other person made a self-disclosure and how it impacted the relationship (positively or negatively)? Was there a reciprocal self-disclosure? If so, did the presence or absence of a reciprocal response enhance the relationship or jeopardize it, and why?*

In most interpersonal communication/relationship scenarios, when one person chooses to self-disclose, the other party in the dyad is expected to reciprocate. However, in health care, patients are asked to self-disclose as part of the information seeking in almost every provider–patient interaction. However, although patients are expected to self-disclose, providers are discouraged from reciprocating. This is antithetical to the norm in our culture and what is expected in all other aspects of interpersonal communication/relationships. As a consequence, it is important for providers to understand how unique this situation is for patients and to use empathic listening to be supportive of patients when they self-disclose difficult or painful information and not just treat the situation as if it is normative for the patient.

Skills Exercise

Talk with someone you know well and stand up to talk when she or he is sitting. How does it make you feel not being at eye level? Next, with a different friend or loved one, have a pad of paper or a smartphone or electronic tablet, and while talking to the person, start looking at and/or writing/typing on the paper or e-device. How does that impact your ability to focus on what the other person is saying? Ask the person how he or she perceived the communication based on your behaviors?

Video Discussion Exercise

Analyze the video

- *The Doctor* (1991)

Role-Play Using These Interactive Simulation Exercises

Pagano, M. (2015). *Communication case studies for health care professionals: An applied approach* (2nd ed.). New York, NY: Springer Publishing Company.

- Chapter 5, "Autonomy Is a Myth" (pp. 45–54)
- Chapter 7, "Closings" (pp. 67–78)
- Chapter 20, "The Nurses Paid More Attention to the Computer Than They Did to Me" (pp. 201–208)

Health Care Issues in the Media

A doctor's story
http://well.blogs.nytimes.com/2015/06/25/sharing-my-story-with-patients/?smid=nytcore-ipad-share&smprod=nytcore-ipad

A nurse's story
http://well.blogs.nytimes.com/2013/09/13/when-nurses-bond-with-their-patients

Health Communication Outcomes

Provider health communication at its most basic level is interpersonal. It is fundamentally diverse, dyadic interaction between providers and patients and/or providers and providers. However, interpersonal communication is generally, in American culture, intended to help develop and/or maintain interpersonal relationships. In health care, however, because of the scientific/biomedical approach of many providers, interpersonal communication becomes more monologue-like, with a paternalistic and authoritarian style that includes health care jargon/terminology, a detective-like inquisition during which patients are peppered with closed-ended questions that serve to verbally and nonverbally demonstrate the provider-centered nature of the interaction. This unique communication style used by many health care professionals is intended to primarily gather the material the provider needs and/or share information that the provider controls. These verbal and nonverbal behaviors also serve to reinforce the provider's role and goals, frequently without any effort to assure that these are shared or mutually constructed patient-centered goals. Furthermore, with a disease-focused approach, it becomes even easier for many providers to neglect the impact that gender, not just sex, has on both communication and health care issues. The importance of assessing a patient's gendered communication preferences, as well as offering carefully considered verbal and nonverbal provider behaviors, can help health care professionals be more effective in their interactions based on the patient's messages and masculine- versus feminine-gendered communication behaviors.

■ REFERENCES

Hall, E. (1959). *The silent language.* New York, NY: Random House.

U.S. Department of Education, National Center for Education Statistics. (2015). *National assessment of adult literacy.* Retrieved from http://nces.ed.gov/naal/kf_demographics.asp

U.S. Department of Education, National Institute on Literacy. (2015). *U.S. Illiteracy statistics.* Retrieved from http://www.statisticbrain.com/number-of-american-adults-who-cant-read

Wood, J. T. (2015). *Gendered lives: Communication, gender, and culture* (11th ed.). Stamford, CT: Cengage Learning.

■ BIBLIOGRAPHY

Korsch, B., & Negrete, V. (1972). Doctor-patient communication. *Scientific American, 227,* 66–74.

Lederman, L. (2008). *Beyond these walls: Readings in health communication.* New York, NY: Oxford University Press.

Ratzan, S. (1994). Health communication as negotiation: The Healthy America Act. *American Behavioral Scientist, 38,* 224–247.

Servellen, G. (2009). *Communication skills for the health care professional: Concepts, practice, and evidence* (2nd ed.). Sudbury, MA: Jones & Bartlett.

Tongue, J., Epps, H., & Forese, L. (2005). Communication skills for patient-centered care. *Journal of Bone and Joint Surgery, 87,* 652–658.

Trenholm, S., & Jensen, A. (2013). *Interpersonal communication* (7th ed.). New York, NY: Oxford University Press.

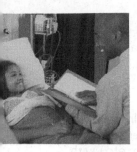

CHAPTER 4

Provider–Patient Communication

For the purpose of this text, we are going to use the following as working definitions:

- *Active listening:* Showing the other person in an interaction that you are listening through nonverbal cues like nodding, eye contact, and/or leaning toward the speaker; and by giving verbal feedback (restating what was heard, or by asking questions to assure accuracy)

- *Audience analysis:* Assessing the other person in an interaction to determine his or her first language, literacy, and education level—both verbal and written—in order to properly tailor a message to meet that person's needs, expectations, and abilities to assimilate the information communicated

- *Closed-ended questions:* Queries intended to gain specific responses, "How long have you had a cough?" or "Are you coughing up something?" or "How high was your fever?" Generally used to limit the feedback from the respondent and to obtain specific information sought by the communicator

- *Empowerment:* Providing patients with information they can use to participate in their health care decision making

- *Narratives:* The stories patients respond with in answer to open-ended questions, such as, "How are you doing?" or "How are you feeling today?"

- *Open-ended questions:* Inquiries that encourage narratives—expanded responses—not short answers

■ NARRATIVES

In American culture we use storytelling—narratives—to make sense of the world. We begin by reading and telling stories to infants about their parents, siblings, the family history, and so forth. We use oral histories and photos from books to inform and engage. Throughout all aspects of American life, stories are used make sense of our lives. One of the major uses of narratives is discussing health issues with friends and family.

Reflection 4.1. Think of a recent sickness, an upper respiratory illness (URI), sometimes called a "cold," or a sore throat, and so forth. When you were discussing how you felt and how your life was impacted (work, school, plans, etc.) with a friend or family member, how did you describe what you were experiencing or had experienced? Be as detailed as possible in your recounting of your part of the conversation.

_____

_____

_____

_____

_____

So, the narrative discussion of your signs and symptoms is typical of most interpersonal communication between individuals in a dyadic discussion. For example, it generally is not atypical to hear two friends discuss an illness as follows:

Jill: "Hi, how are you doing? I missed you in calculus today."

Jean: "I am so sick."

Jill: "What's up?"

Jean: "I woke up last night soaked in sweat, I felt like I was burning up. And my throat hurt so bad when I swallowed that I couldn't even drink water."

Jill: "Did you go to the health center?"

Jean: "No, I took some Motrin and some throat things my mom had packed for me when I moved in, they helped, and I got some sleep—didn't even wake up until after class. I don't think I have a fever, but my throat is still sore and my nose is all plugged up. Think I should go to the health center?"

Reflection 4.2. Think about the last time you went to a health care provider for an acute illness or injury. What happened when you tried to tell your story/narrative? Did the provider allow you to describe it as you wanted? Or did he or she stop you (interrupt) with questions? If the latter, how did the interruptions make you feel about the information exchange with your provider?

_____

_____

_____

_____

_____

In this example, Jean is telling her story, Jill only interrupts to inquire whether she has sought medical care—an interpersonal, empathic-listening query about her friend's illness. However, Jean not only wants to tell her story, she wants to explain more about her situation to try to allay her friend's concerns and seek some advice. These types of narratives are typical in American culture, especially as they relate to people's desires to share stories about their health and use these narratives to continue to build relationships with close friends and/or family. At the same time, these communicators are trying to gather feedback and input for their own health care assessment and decision making.

If narratives are so expected/important in our culture, how do you think patients feel when they do not get to tell their stories? In 21st-century health care, because of time constraints and the biomedical model, many health care providers use a disease-centric approach. For example, let's assume Jean goes to the health center and, after waiting to see a provider, has the following exchange:

Provider: "Hi, what can I do for you today?"

Jean: "I'm not feeling good."

Provider: "Okay, so do you have a fever?"

Jean: "Yes, and …"

Provider: "How high?"

Jean: "I don't know, I don't have a thermometer in my dorm. But I woke up all sweaty and …"

Provider: "Well, your temp is normal here, are you coughing?"

Jean: "A little, mostly when I lay down. But it's my throat."

Provider: "You sound like your nose is congested, so it's likely a postnasal drip that is causing your cough when you lay down, which irritates your throat, and then you're probably mouth breathing with a stopped up nose, so that would also contribute to your throat irritation. We'll do a strep test to rule out a strep throat, but without a fever, it's likely a virus and you'll need a decongestant, some fluids, and rest. Let me examine you quickly and then we'll get that throat swabbed."

How would you analyze this conversation? Did the provider get the information needed to make a diagnosis? How would you assess the provider's communication from the patient's perspective? If the provider is working from a biomedical approach, he or she is striving to find the cause of this patient's illness and fix it. Using our health communication lens we can assess the provider's behaviors in this example. The provider:

- Gathered information from the patient
- Compared the patient's signs (temperature and vital signs) and symptoms (cough, sore throat, nasal congestion)

- Analyzed findings against an algorithm for viral versus bacterial infections and other possible etiologies based on the patient's complaints

- Decided on a likely course of action/treatment based on questions, physical exam, and strep test

From the provider's goal-attainment perspective, we could argue that he or she got the information needed to arrive at a working diagnosis in a fairly brief amount of time. However, this approach is disease- and provider-centric. It is about what the provider needs to diagnose and treat the illness. However, it does not recognize that the patient may have needs/goals that are not disease/provider focused.

If we assess the provider–patient interaction from Jean's perspective using a health/interpersonal communication lens, we can deduce that the patient was:

- Prevented from communicating her narrative as she would in other parts of her life

- Interrupted numerous times, demonstrating the provider's power and the patient's limited role in the relationship

- Diagnosed, at least provisionally, with minimal information

- Regarded, nonverbally and verbally, differently than she would be in almost any other context in American culture

Therefore, it would not be surprising that the provider's unwillingness to allow Jean to tell her story negatively impacted their provider–patient relationship and consequently lowered Jean's level of trust in the provider's diagnosis, treatment plan, and prognosis. Providers should perceive the simple act of allowing a patient to share his or her narrative, not as a waste of time, but as *both* information-gathering and relationship-building opportunities. The uninterrupted communication of the patient's symptoms permits him or her to feel that the provider respects him or her and that the common act of narrative sharing extends to health communication as well. Furthermore, the patient's ability to share his or her narrative also communicates a provider's willingness to share power vis-à-vis listening, not just controlling the conversation via provider-focused, disease-centered messages.

■ LISTENING VERSUS TALKING

As discussed in Chapter 3, listening is critical to effective interpersonal and health communication. However, not only is listening different from hearing, active listening and empathic listening can also be used to build a relationship, encourage a speaker to share more information, and assure the speaker that the listener is assimilating the material and cares about him or her. For health care providers, especially those who follow a biomedical approach to health care delivery, gathering specific information—related to an algorithm or a disease/injury focus—often leads to providers talking more than listening.

Furthermore, in order to gather the information they want/need, many health care professionals tend to interrupt patients frequently, which is not only the opposite of patient-centered listening, but is typical of masculine-gendered behavior. As well as contributing to a paternalistic perception by patients, interruptions frequently limit patients' interests in sharing and/or opportunities to communicate additional information.

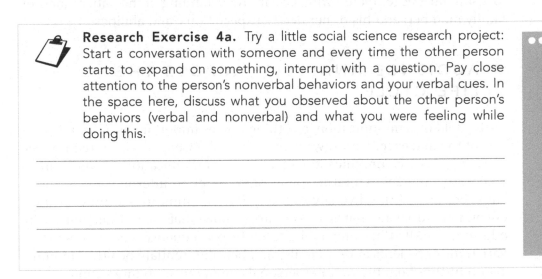

Research Exercise 4a. Try a little social science research project: Start a conversation with someone and every time the other person starts to expand on something, interrupt with a question. Pay close attention to the person's nonverbal behaviors and your verbal cues. In the space here, discuss what you observed about the other person's behaviors (verbal and nonverbal) and what you were feeling while doing this.

For the most part, in American culture, communicators prefer not to be interrupted. Instead one person likes to complete his or her narrative before the other person speaks/interrupts. However, in a disease-focused, provider-centric health care system, the patient's communication needs/desires are often overlooked or undervalued. Furthermore, when a person feels his or her messages/narratives are less important than the other communicator in the dyad, the patient is less likely to want to share information but also less likely to want to engage in interpersonal communication or to develop/maintain an interpersonal relationship. Although it is true, that providers cannot allow patients to endlessly tell their stories, for the most part waiting a minute or two for patients to complete their narratives about their signs (temperature, increased pulse, lump, etc.), symptoms (pain, feeling, nausea, etc.), or events allows them to feel that they shared the information they felt was important and, if the provider truly listens, many, if not most, of the provider's questions will often be answered. And, if not, closed-ended questions

(How high was your fever? or, When did the vomiting start?) can be used to gather more detailed data for diagnosis and treatments. However, using an open-ended question (Tell me why you came in today? or simply, How are you doing?) without interruption will help maintain the larger culture's interpersonal communication expectations for patients. In addition, using open-ended queries to initiate a conversation allows providers to build a relationship by demonstrating the importance of patients' narratives in the provider–patient interaction. Furthermore, the simple act of using an uninterrupted open-ended question to seek information serves to equalize the power in the relationship versus using a paternalistic/autocratic, interrogative interrupting style that nonverbally communicates the provider's power. The value of open-ended, uninterrupted initial information-seeking behaviors still must be tempered with a clear understanding of the patient (and/or family member) and his or her needs, expectations, and abilities.

■ AUDIENCE ANALYSIS: ACROSS THE LIFE CYCLE

In the field of communication, few things are as important as a careful analysis of the audience. Typically, we think of audience analysis more in public speaking, mass communication, or written communication—health care is again very different in interpersonal communication/interpersonal relationships because of the diversity of potential communicators a provider may encounter—from neonates to comatose individuals and from minimally educated to MD/PhD-prepared adults. In consequence, the demographic variations of patients and/or family members differentiate health communication further from typical interpersonal communication interactions.

Reflection 4.3. Consider your close friends and family—those you have interpersonal communication/relationships with (know well and share common goals with). How would not knowing how educated they were or what their prior experiences in a similar relationship might have been impact how you communicate with them?

_____

_____

_____

_____

_____

For example, in terms of how you communicate, if you are going to talk to an 8-year-old child, does it matter if he or she has a cold or a tumor? Or will you speak with the child the same way regardless? Similarly, if you are speaking with an adult patient who does not have a college education, how would that impact your conversation? As you likely have noticed, the possible differences between patients and/or family members are as diverse and expansive as the U.S. population. The specific impact of health literacy and stereotyping will be discussed later in this chapter, but let's focus our thoughts on the value of audience analysis related to several other key patient demographic areas:

- Age
  - Pediatric
  - Adolescent
  - Adult
  - Geriatric
- Education
  - Speaking
  - Reading
  - Assimilating
- Sex
- Gender
- Socioeconomic status (SES)

■ AGE

One of the many aspects of health care that differentiates it from most other aspects of our lives in terms of interpersonal communication has to do with the differences in demographics between providers and their patients. Few adults have interpersonal communication/relationships with young children (except with their own); however, in many health care roles and professions it is not uncommon for providers to need to communicate with children of all ages. And depending on the context for the child's illness/injury/visit, he or she may be the most important source of information. Therefore, it is critical to analyze how to best communicate with the child patient and/or parent. If possible, it is wise to acknowledge the patient/child first, then the parent. Too often, for speed, or ease of information gathering, the parent is the focus of the provider's communication and attention. When this approach is taken by providers, especially in emergency departments (EDs) and nonpediatric practices, the context takes on more of a veterinary exam with the child being there for the exam and the parent being the source of almost all information. A few simple steps can help the child be more trusting and want to share in the process.

For example, you might want to sit at the child's level, ask about school, pets, or siblings to try and demonstrate your interest in what she or he has to say. Be just as cognizant of your nonverbal behaviors with pediatric patients as you are with adults; if the child is old enough, offer to shake his or her hand, ask before touching/examining the patient, and explain what you are going to do before you do it. Try to learn about the child's prior health communication experiences—did he or she have ED visits, hospitalizations, or other unusual or "traumatic" health care experiences? Remember, communication is *continuous*, so you want to make this as positive an experience as possible (for the current as well as future encounters with you and other providers). At the same time, recognizing and acknowledging a past problematic or painful health care experience up front and trying to explain how this visit will be different is an effort toward easing some of the patient's and parents' concerns and may possibly change the dynamic from fear and mistrust to a willingness to contribute to the success of the interaction. However, not unlike many other aspects of the life cycle, providers must be aware of how easy it is to ignore or minimize input from older patients as well.

Research Exercise 4b. Why not try to apply this approach to pediatric interactions and do a brief research project. Find a child, a 5- to 10-year-old, not a member of your family or a patient and, with his or her parent's permission, introduce yourself and ask the child to tell you about school, toys, books, whatever he or she wants to discuss and listen to what the child says and see how easily you can begin to have a conversation about the topic. In this space, describe what you learned about communicating interpersonally with a child and how that might be useful to you in your professional role when examining/treating/caring for a pediatric patient.

_____

_____

_____

_____

_____

Rather than move chronologically in our discussion of the role age plays in effective health communication exchanges, let's discuss the opposite end of the life cycle. How do you see interacting with geriatric patients being similar to or different from pediatric patient communication? Not unlike health care visits with children, many providers tend to communicate with family members or caregivers rather than with elderly patients. With our aging population, adults older than 60 now make up a large portion of the patient population. Therefore, it is much more common to see 80-, 90-, and 100-year-olds in both acute and chronic care settings, not just in long-term care facilities. As a consequence, audience analysis for advanced-aged patients should include their level of acuity (both for communication and clinical perspectives) and, whenever possible, the provider should be elder-patient focused and not family member/caregiver-centric. As in pediatric interactions, the provider needs to determine the best nonverbal and verbal actions to utilize to demonstrate his or her interest in communicating with the geriatric patient; overall a few approaches to consider include:

- Nonverbal behaviors
  - Paralinguistic cues
    - Volume—may need to be higher than usual, depending on the patient's hearing acuity
    - Tone—conversational, not paternalistic or condescending
    - Speed—may need to slow down your talking
  - Careful attention to patient's feedback/assimilation
  - Haptics—as with others, touch appropriately and with permission
  - Kinesics—try to sit at eye level, pay more attention to the patient than to the computer or family member/caregiver
  - Proxemics—consider sitting closer to the patient if that improves his or her hearing/assimilation/exchange of information
  - Written communication—language (educational and ethnic) appropriate, font size as needed for patient's visual acuity, and with clear instructions for how to follow up with unanswered questions (phone, e-mail, office visit, etc.)
- Verbal behaviors
  - Interpersonal—strive to use expected communication messages
    - Introductions
    - Goal setting
    - Feedback
    - Next steps
    - Educational, mental acuity, and appropriate language choices

Although end-of-life discussions are important throughout adulthood, based on the context of the geriatric patient–provider interaction, it is important to discuss advance directives and living-will issues with senior citizens. If they have already made these decisions, it will only take a few minutes to determine that, but if they have not, this is a critically important educational opportunity for providers talking with geriatric patients. As this may be an emotionally charged issue, the patient may want a family member present to also hear the information, and it is critically important to have written material for the patient and family member/caregiver to take with them to review later in a less intense context. Until the provider is certain that the patient has been fully informed and able to reach a decision about living-will and/or advance directive issues—this topic should be a part of all follow-up interactions. Although there are similarities in the communication challenges associated with provider–patient interactions with pediatric and geriatric individuals—there are also concerns related specifically to adolescent and adult health communication.

Although the issues related to health communication with pediatric and geriatric patients may seem more obvious, many providers have nearly as many interpersonal communication/relationship difficulties with adolescent and/or adult patients. As you may have surmised, for a variety of reasons (emotional, hormonal, social, etc.), adolescents present a unique set of potential communication-related problems. Adolescents frequently do not want to discuss or feel uncomfortable discussing personal issues with adults (parents and health care providers). Similarly, many providers feel awkward having health-related conversations with adolescents. The fact that these young men and women are literally in between childhood and adulthood makes them both emotionally sensitive, hormonally challenged, and physically evolving. As a consequence, from a communication perspective, it becomes a question of when to treat them as adults (verbally and nonverbally)? For example, at what age should the patient decide whether a parent should be in the exam room for nonlife-threatening, provider–patient interactions? When does a provider need a chaperone and should that be part of the office/hospital/clinic staff's job or the parent's?

Reflection 4.4. Think back to when you were 14 or 15, how did you feel about communicating when you went to see your health care provider? Did you want to have a dyadic interaction or did you want a parent involved? How about when it came time for the examination? Did you want your parent present or not? How do you think these feelings impacted your willingness to communicate with the provider (ask/answer questions, gather information, etc.)?

From a communication perspective, it would seem ideal if the patient (adolescent) could decide whether his or her parent was in the conversation and/or exam with the provider. However, until children are 18 parents legally have the right to be involved in all aspects of their children's care. Therefore, a provider may want to explain to both the parent and the adolescent child at the first visit that because the patient is getting older he or she may want to have a bit more privacy with the provider. If you are going to use a chaperone (especially for exams) you would want to make that clear as well. Then let the parent and child negotiate whether the parent stays or not—this way the adolescent knows that the provider recognizes her or him as more an independent adult than a pediatric patient. From an interpersonal communication/relationship-building perspective, it should help establish the provider's intention to treat the adolescent as much like an adult as possible. Consequently, regardless of whether the parent remains or leaves, the provider needs to be patient-centric in his or her communication and only include the parent as needed for clarity, or as demanded by the mother or father. It is important to constantly remind yourself that the nonverbal communication of disinterest and limited verbal responses are typical for adolescent–adult interactions regardless of the context. However, the more your verbal and nonverbal behaviors demonstrate your interest in the adolescent and helping him or her stay healthy vis-à-vis your verbal and nonverbal behaviors, the more likely you are to eventually build a trusting interpersonal relationship and increase the opportunity for information sharing and mutual goal attainment. One of the key opportunities for adolescent–provider health communication is often also a formidable challenge—assuring patients are educated about sexual behaviors, pregnancy risks, and sexually transmitted diseases. Providers need to assess what their adolescent patients know about these critically important health communication topics and evaluate the most effective way to help educate and empower these young adults. Although face-to-face (F2F) discussions and feedback are generally ideal, age-, language-, and literacy-appropriate written communication/handouts are often a good way to encourage a dialogue. Providing the materials and allowing some time for the adolescent to read them before having a discussion is ideal, but this may not always be practical. Therefore, providers need to analyze the adolescent and the context to determine the best way to educate the patient and use feedback to determine assimilation, confusion, and/or misperceptions. However, providers should ask adolescents what they know about sex, where they got their information, and correct any misinformation—as well as encourage these patients to always feel free to discuss the topic at any time they have questions or a health concern. Assuring them of confidentiality will likely be another opportunity to build trust and an interpersonal relationship. Conversations about sex and a patient's sexual history are just one aspect of the provider–patient interaction from adolescence through adulthood.

As patients age, especially if they have continuity of care from adolescence into adulthood, it will be easier to maintain and enhance an interpersonal relationship. As with any relationship over time, generally there is an increase in trust and in health communication a heightened exchange of information and patient self-disclosure. Therefore, it is important for providers to use effective interpersonal and gendered communication (see Chapter 3) in an effort to further the relationship and improve information sharing, power sharing, and empowered decision making. As will be discussed further, it is critically important for providers to recognize the problems associated with stereotyping (addiction, sexual orientation, etc.) and how such behaviors limit information exchanges, analysis, and effective health communication/outcomes. However, providers also need to recognize that audience analysis needs to also include demographics beyond age, such as the patient's education level.

■ EDUCATION

Although some demographics are more obvious, or even documented (sex or age), a person's education may not be as clear. For example, according to the U.S. Department of Education and the National Institute of Literacy, nearly 15% of adult Americans cannot read, and over 20% cannot read at the fifth-grade level. Therefore, consider many of the communication behaviors we treat as commonplace today: filling out health care forms, following preoperative/postoperative instructions, understanding educational pamphlets/brochures, or even prescription labels. How do you think these educational deficiencies might impact the provider–patient information exchange?

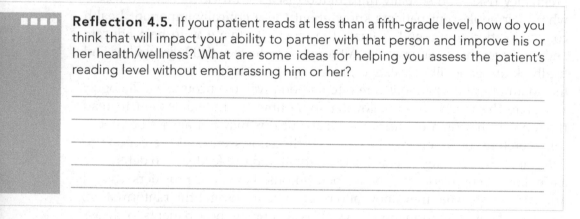

Reflection 4.5. If your patient reads at less than a fifth-grade level, how do you think that will impact your ability to partner with that person and improve his or her health/wellness? What are some ideas for helping you assess the patient's reading level without embarrassing him or her?

And literacy, though often categorized solely by reading, from a health communication perspective really does include not just verbal, written, and reading aspects, but assimilation ability as well. Health literacy will be discussed in more detail later in this chapter, but it is important for providers to recognize the interdependent nature of these disparate but interrelated behaviors. For example, if a patient cannot read a health form, she or he will likely not relate all the information the provider needs. In addition, if the patient cannot verbally communicate effectively and/or is unable to assimilate the provider's messages because of literacy issues, the interaction will not only be frustrating for all, but may in fact, be useless or, in the worst possible scenario, dangerous as the patient misunderstands the treatment plan, instructions, and so on. The importance of analyzing patients' abilities to read, assimilate, and communicate/share information are critical to the communication/collaboration of patients and providers. And the very troubling reality is that if someone speaks a foreign language it is generally easy for a provider to recognize that and seek a professional translator. However, if the patient seemingly speaks the same language as the provider, without some careful analysis, it may be very difficult for the provider to determine not only the patient's education level, but his or her verbal, reading, and assimilating abilities. Although the analysis of a patient's education (reading, speaking, and assimilating) often needs careful scrutiny, the role of sex in provider–patient communication is more obvious, but still frequently underassessed and/or underappreciated.

■ SEX

Although age has a breadth of communication-related issues that need to be analyzed by a provider, the patient's sex and how it impacts the delivery of health care needs to be similarly assessed. Much has been made about the differences in the communication styles of males and females, especially in health care settings. Again, providers need to be aware of this potential but not consider it a stereotype. Therefore, because it has been postulated that males tend to provide less information and ask fewer questions than females, providers need to make sure that they are seeking feedback and using a variety of formats (verbal and nonverbal/written) to try to gain information from patients of both sexes. The provider needs to use effective interpersonal communication to build relationships with patients regardless of their sex and to assure that the patient is given time to not only share his or her narrative, but ask questions, clarify misperceptions, and/or be encouraged to fully discuss his or her health/illness/injury issues. Similar to assessing the patient's sex in terms of health communication approaches, the provider should also consider the patient's gender.

■ GENDER

As discussed in Chapter 3, gender communication is often difficult to analyze but critically important to how individuals communicate. Therefore, it is essential for providers to not stereotype patients based on their sex (male = masculine and/or female = feminine), but to analyze their gendered behaviors to enhance the information sharing and interpersonal communication/relationship possibilities. Clearly, a person's gendered communication often makes a difference in how he or she not only shares information, but seeks care, follows up, and/or trusts the provider.

Generally speaking, feminine-gendered individuals (male or female), tend to ask more questions, share more detailed information, seek feedback, and interrupt less than masculine-gendered communicators (male or female). Therefore, it should not be surprising that individuals who want to provide detailed information and discuss their feelings, not just their signs and symptoms, are often perceived as potential hypochondriacs or hormonally imbalanced. In fact, it may be that many of these patients were feminine gendered and wanted to provide more information, encourage a discussion, participate

Research Exercise 4c. Consider two people you know but preferably with whom you are not "close friends" who behave the opposite of what might be expected in this culture from a gender perspective; a male who communicates with a more feminine-gendered style and a female who has a more masculine-gendered communication behavior. Independently, ask each to tell you a story about his or her childhood (anything they want) and try to note not just the content of the story, but the amount of detail, the interest in sharing it with you versus any reluctance or even refusal, and so forth. What did you learn about how gender impacts information sharing and how stereotyping gender based on sex might be problematic for you as a health care provider?

_____

_____

_____

_____

_____

and collaborate in their treatment decision making, and so forth. Similarly, males are often characterized, even stereotyped, as not wanting to go to health care providers, offer much information, or ask questions and yet many of those masculine-gendered behaviors are the same ones that are not only expected but are praised in professional organizations. The more competitive, independent, and aggressive the professional, regardless of the career, the more he or she attempts to be in control, self-serving, and taking a leadership role. Therefore, health care providers must seek ways to encourage patients—based on their gendered behaviors/communication—to not only seek information, but share it, and participate in the decision making, treatment plans, and thus enhance their health/wellness outcomes. Although a patient's age, education, sex, and gender can and should be analyzed in terms of communication effectiveness, the impact of similar or different SES on provider–patient interactions needs to also be analyzed and addressed.

Reflection 4.6. What are some of the communication behaviors you can observe in order to help analyze a patient's gender? How might you use your findings to enhance your interaction with the patient if the patient is masculine versus feminine gendered?

_____

_____

_____

_____

_____

■ SOCIOECONOMIC STATUS

The role of SES in provider–patient communication is somewhat different than the other demographics that providers analyze. Understanding the potential impact of SES on patient–provider interactions is very important. Humans frequently use their perceptions of similarity with another communicator to determine how much they are alike and therefore the more comparable they may be in values and beliefs. Consequently, many patients assess providers based on their SES and how similar/dissimilar they are. Therefore, in U.S. culture, it should not be surprising that most patients will assume that providers are quite different from themselves—educationally, economically, and socially. Although providers clearly cannot change their SES based on the patient, being aware of the potential impact of SES on provider–patient communication, relationship development, and trust building can help you use interpersonal communication that minimizes the differences between you and your patient and maximizes your desire to partner with him or her and attain the goal of improving/maintaining his or her health/wellness.

The point of assessing the role SES differences might have in provider–patient communication is to help you further understand that just because the provider asks a question, or communicates what may be a very carefully considered plan of action, does not mean it will be similarly perceived that way by another communicator. For example, if you think a patient needs to lose weight, eat a more healthy diet, and exercise more—those may all be very accurate assessments and plans to improve the patient's health. However, a health care provider who likely is in the upper middle or upper class in American culture generally is not perceived to have any problem purchasing food or shelter. That economic assumption is part of the SES that creates conflict for many patients. Eating healthier, for example, is a wonderful plan—as long as someone can afford it. But if a patient only has $1.50 for dinner, a fast-food burger or taco is going to be the most likely choice. Therefore, although providers have been

Reflection 4.7. Recall a time when you felt someone (preferably not a health care provider) you were communicating with had a different socioeconomic status (SES) than you—perhaps as a student with a professor, or as a college intern, or with a summer employer, and so forth. How did that difference in SES, the dissimilarity you perceived between yourself and the other person, impact how you felt about him or her and your willingness to communicate any more than was required?

_____

_____

_____

_____

_____

trained in nutrition, exercise physiology, and weight control, these topics are of very little importance to a patient who is making decisions about whether to eat or pay rent, or eat or buy prescriptions.

SES analysis then is important in helping providers recognize how they can best help their patients—not just provide accurate information, but collaborate in developing plans that can be realistically managed by the patient based on his or her social and economic situation. By not assuming that all patients can manage their health equally from a SES perspective, providers demonstrate to their patients that they may not share the same status, but recognize the differences among all Americans and the desire to find ways to provide health care options that are appropriate given the patient's current SES. However, part of this awareness of the role SES plays in health care delivery and provider–patient communication requires that providers not stereotype patients based on their artifacts (clothes, hairdo, jewelry, body art, etc.). Like SES, stereotyping can create more barriers to effective health and interpersonal communication and relationship development.

■ STEREOTYPES AND MARGINALIZED POPULATIONS

As previously mentioned, stereotyping and a provider's potential bias toward marginalized populations (e.g., addicts, the homeless, grossly obese, mentally impaired, and elderly) can markedly limit effective health and interpersonal communication. Clearly, there is a likely relationship between stereotyping and marginalized populations that can be increased based on the provider's prior experiences, social and psychological biases, and provider–provider/peer pressure. It is very important, however, for health care professionals to analyze not just the communication needs of patients who might be perceived from a stereotypical or marginalized perspective, but also intrapersonally—from the provider's perspective. Although experience

Reflection 4.8. Picture a 35-year-old patient in your emergency department (ED) who just crashed his motorcycle; he is complaining of pain from his broken right foot and badly abraded left forearm. From a psychological/sociological perspective, what do you see when you look at him? Be as detailed as possible. What do you hypothesize is his profession and why?

_____

_____

_____

_____

_____

can inform the provider's decision making and information sharing as well as diagnosis and treatment plans, it is important to remember that just because a prior patient(s) behaved a certain way, does not mean that all patients with similar problems, behaviors, needs, and so forth should be treated like the prior patient(s). Spending less time communicating with a patient because of conclusions the provider has made based on stereotyping or marginalized population biases is not only unfair to the individual patient, but unethical, and, on some level, is likely dangerous (medically and/or legally). The more providers can analyze the health care problems, needs, expectations, and communication behaviors/messages of the individual patient he or she is interacting with in a social vacuum, the more effective the information exchange is likely to be and the more potentially beneficial the interpersonal communication/relationship will be for both communicators. This approach is not to suggest that the experiences and knowledge of the provider should not help inform the communication and collaboration with the patient, but that is far different than dismissing the patient as lazy, unwilling to work, an addict who has no desire to change, or hopeless. Taking a quick minute to analyze not just the patient, but your own response to the patient will provide invaluable information for not only your communication, but also your ability to actively listen, assimilate, and assess the patient's situation based on the data, not on bias or presumption. This notion of not assuming/presuming is important to avoid stereotyping and bias against marginalized populations, but also to assessing the health literacy of your audience/patients.

■ HEALTH LITERACY

Although most patients do not attempt to hide their sex, or even their age and education, patients with lower health literacy may either not realize it, or be unwilling or embarrassed to admit it. Therefore, it is often best to assume that patients have limited health literacy and be sure that your verbal and written messages are not only communicated in non–health care terms, but also at fifth- or sixth-grade reading levels. However, as mentioned earlier, the only way to be sure that patients are able to understand your messages, assimilate the information, and use it to make decisions is to use feedback via questions to assess what the other communicator heard, read, and comprehended. Analyzing your patient's health literacy would also be aided by asking him or her to read a few sentences or a short paragraph, to determine his or her literacy in general, as well as the patient's ability to interpret the message. Finally, you could also include a typical prescription text (e.g., take one tablet every other day; avoid alcohol and citrus fruit) and ask the patient to tell you what specific days he or she will be taking the medicine and what else the patient needs to do according to the prescription—remember, this is not about repeating the words on the prescription, but how the patient interprets the meaning of those words. For example, what does the patient think "avoid alcohol" means (e.g., just liquor, or also wine and beer, or does he think "rubbing alcohol")? And can the patient tell you which fruits are "citrus"? These simple cognitive tests can become a standard part of your evaluation, in which case you are assessing literacy and comprehension as part of your mental health and neurologic exam—not to embarrass the patient but to help gather data about the patient's overall wellness and health. For example, you could use a fifth-grade-reading-level example from a credible source, like this one from the North Carolina State University, William & Ida Friday Institute for Educational Innovation, and ask the patient to read it aloud:

Hurricanes

Hurricanes are large tropical storms that develop in the oceans of the world. Hurricanes gather heat and energy from the warm ocean water. The heat from these warm currents increases the power of the hurricane. Hurricanes that remain over warm water usually get bigger and stronger, but they weaken once they get over land. Hurricanes are storms that are given names, and a new list of names is created each year. The first hurricane name starts with the letter A, like Ashley, and the names move through the alphabet as more hurricanes form. (North Carolina State University, 2006)

 Research Exercise 4d. Ask a variety of friends and strangers to explain to you what the term *avoid alcohol* (liquor, beer, wine, combinations of any of these) means to them. Then ask them to name as many "citrus fruits" (grapefruit, lemons, limes, oranges, tangerines) as they can? How did your data collection confirm or conflict with your hypotheses about who would be able to most effectively answer these questions? And how does that relate to audience analysis, stereotyping, and health literacy?

After the patient reads the paragraph, you could ask the patient to tell you how hurricanes are named, where they develop, or how they are formed. In this way, you can both listen to the patient's ability to read at a fifth-grade level, but also assess his or her comprehension of the material to assure not just reading ability, but literacy/understanding.

This chapter has focused on many aspects of provider–patient communication. It is important to remember that the goal of this text is to help providers become more effective interpersonal and health communicators by taking a patient-centric, relationship-building approach to provider–patient interactions. Therefore, in this chapter we have discussed the value of narratives, listening versus talking, and audience analysis across patients' life cycles. In addition, the value of recognizing the impact of various demographics, SES, and health literacy on health communication effectiveness and relationship building cannot be overemphasized.

Reflections (among the possible responses)

4.1. Think of a recent sickness, an upper respiratory illness (URI), sometimes called a "cold," or a sore throat, and so forth. When you were discussing how you felt and how your life was impacted (work, school, plans, etc.) with a friend or family member, how did you describe what you were experiencing or had experienced? Be as detailed as possible in your recounting of your part of the conversation.

When most Americans describe a life event, it is not done with a bulleted statement but instead a detailed narrative that includes both factual and emotional data. For example, if you were telling a friend or parent about a recent URI, it would likely be similar to this scenario:

You: "Mom, I think I have some kind of cold or flu. I woke up during the night and my bed was soaked; I just hurt all over. My legs ached so bad, I didn't know if I could stand up. And then I got back to sleep, but when I got up this morning my nose was stopped up and my throat hurts, and I am so tired."

This narrative is not just a list of symptoms:

- Sweat
- Myalgias (muscle aches)
- Nasal congestion
- Pharyngeal irritation (sore throat)
- Malaise (tired)

but instead a detailed discussion of both physical complaints and emotional feelings. Although most health care providers want the symptoms, bulleted previously, the brief extra verbiage in a narrative provides the same data, but just in the patient's normative information-sharing/conversational/interpersonal communication style. It would be very beneficial for providers to recognize the value of narrative use by patients—who feel they were able to "tell their stories" in their usual way—and through which providers get information that they can further refine via closed-ended questions.

4.2. Think about the last time you went to a health care provider for an acute illness or injury. What happened when you tried to tell your story/narrative? Did the provider allow you to describe it as you wanted? Or did he or she stop you (interrupt) with questions? If the latter, how did the interruptions make you feel about the information exchange with your provider?

If your health care provider was utilizing a biomedical approach to information gathering, as many practitioners in this country do, then he or she likely asked a question and as soon as you provided a symptom, the provider interrupted your answer and began using closed-ended questions to gain data that could be used for the algorithm needed to determine your most likely diagnosis/problem. So fever, sore throat, nasal congestion equals URI/virus versus strep throat/bacterial infection with posterior pharyngeal irritation from a postnasal drip as the most likely etiology. Although a series of closed-ended questions to rule out pneumonia, sinusitis, bronchitis, and so forth will be used, the provider relies on the patient's initial information to help determine the organ systems that appear to be impacted by an illness or injury and what algorithm to use in analyzing the etiology, diagnosis, and treatment plan. The key is to recall that the more you can make the patient feel he or she is contributing to/collaborating in the process and sharing the information he or she feels is important for the provider to know, the more effective the communication exchange and interpersonal relationship development will be perceived.

4.3. Consider your close friends and family—those you have impersonal communication/relationships with (know well and share common goals with). How would not knowing how educated they were or what their prior experiences in a similar relationship might have been impact how you communicate with them?

The more we know about a person, the more it enhances an interpersonal platonic, professional, or romantic relationship. For example, if you do not know a person's education level you may use language he or she does not understand or appear condescending in your explanations. Similarly, not knowing a person's education level could create conflict if you assume the person can read at a certain level and that is untrue. One of the realities of American relationships is that we tend to associate with people who we perceive as similar to us—related to age, education, and SES. Therefore, part of the general relationship development process is learning about the other person's background, family, education, and so forth. But this process generally takes place over a prolonged time frame, days, weeks, months, even years. However, in health care, providers and patients generally have minutes to learn about the other person and for patients there is often very little or no opportunity to discover much about the provider's background except from diplomas on the wall or by his or her professional title/degree. As a consequence, the more a provider can try to learn about a patient's education and SES background, the more information the provider will have to analyze how most effectively to communicate with the patient.

4.4. Think back to when you were 14 or 15, how did you feel about communicating when you went to see your health care provider? Did you want to have a dyadic interaction or did you want a parent involved? How about when it came time for the examination? Did you want your parent present or not? How do you think these feelings impacted your willingness to communicate with the provider (ask/answer questions, gather information, etc.)?

Generally, adolescents are reluctant to talk openly with adults and some would prefer to have their parents present while talking with providers and others would prefer to speak independently with their health care professional. Therefore, it would be best if the patient could decide; however, parents are legal guardians and have the right to be present if they so desire. Consequently, although a provider can suggest that an adolescent decide who is present—it is ultimately up to the parent. Regardless, providers should try to make the adolescent the focus of the conversation and seek to encourage a dialogue and information sharing with the patient, not the parent, if possible. The more an adolescent trusts a provider, the more likely he or she will feel comfortable discussing health care issues, asking questions, and participating in his or her treatment plans. And although it is likely wise, ethically and legally, to have a chaperone during physical exams of patients of the opposite sex, providers should certainly be aware of the importance of having a chaperone during an adolescent's examination and have the patient determine (if possible) whether he or she prefers a parent or a health care provider.

4.5. If your patient reads at less than a fifth-grade level, how do you think that will impact your ability to partner with that person and improve his or her health/wellness? What are some ideas for helping you assess the patient's reading level without embarrassing him or her?

As discussed earlier, a patient's reading level impacts his or her health and communication in a number of ways. First, if patients have reading difficulties, they may not be able to appropriately complete the basic office/hospital forms—consequently, the information, even the demographics, could be inaccurate. Second, if patients are embarrassed about their reading literacy, they may not want to disclose that and may even lie to keep it hidden from the provider. Third, if patients have a low literacy level, they will likely have low health literacy as well. Consequently, providers may not be able to use their standard educational handouts, pre- and postprocedure instructions, or prescription labeling. The impact of diminished literacy (reading and health) on health communication information exchange is enormous and can only be improved by providers taking the time to assess a patient's literacy and providing appropriate materials for the patient's reading and health literacy levels. Finally, the provider can use a reading sample (see example given earlier) as part of the patients' exams, to assess their reading levels, as well as their abilities to assimilate and analyze what was read.

4.6. What are some of the communication behaviors you can observe in order to help analyze a patient's gender? How might you use your findings to enhance your interaction with the patient if the patient is masculine versus feminine gendered?

Patients can be observed to determine how they use communication to demonstrate their aggressiveness, independence, competitiveness, or how they want to participate, collaborate, or contribute. Armed with this information, a provider can assess how much to encourage a patient to tell his or her narrative—for more feminine-gendered individuals, or seek more information if a more masculine-gendered patient is averse to discussing his or her pain, problems, and concerns with a provider.

4.7. Recall a time when you felt someone (preferably not a health care provider) you were communicating with had a different socioeconomic status (SES) than you—perhaps as a student with a professor, or as a college intern, or with a summer employer, and so forth. How did that difference in SES, the dissimilarity you perceived between yourself and the other person, impact how you felt about him or her and your willingness to communicate any more than was required?

Often when a person has a different SES from another, especially in an interpersonal relationship, like student–professor, employee–employer, or provider–patient, it will directly impact how comfortable the lower SES person is with information sharing. It may be hard for that person to identify with the higher SES person's role, lifestyle, and so forth. For example, in a conversation with a professor about where to eat off campus, many students might feel awkward because the professor has a higher SES and can choose from a much wider offering of restaurants, from economic, ethnic, and geographic perspectives. Consequently, students would likely not choose to engage with the professor about where to eat, as they don't want to be reminded of the differences in their SES. Similarly, patients may be reluctant to discuss problems or treatment options with providers if they feel the differences in their SES will make it impossible for the provider to understand their predicament—for example, the patient cannot afford time off work, more nutritious meals, or the price of certain medications. Providers need to recognize the potential patient issues related to SES differences in order to not appear elitist, aloof, or uncaring.

4.8. Picture a 35-year-old patient in your emergency department (ED) who just crashed his motorcycle; he is complaining of pain from his broken right foot and badly abraded left forearm. From a psychological/sociological perspective, what do you see when you look at him? Be as detailed as possible. What do you hypothesize is his profession and why?

Working in an ED and seeing injuries from motorcycle accidents, providers have to guard against stereotyping every person who rides a motorcycle as being careless, a risk taker, or a member of a motorcycle gang. Lots of people are in automobile accidents and for the most part they generally are not judged as reckless or in a gang based on their choice of a car for transportation. Stereotypes only serve to bias the provider, limit the information exchange, and potentially alienate the patient and/or negatively impact his or her care. Instead of trying to judge a patient's behaviors, it would be more productive and patient centered to focus on the injuries, diagnosis, information exchange, and treatment plan. It is very important to remind yourself that health care providers, judges, lawyers, and countless other professionals ride motorcycles. Therefore, it makes no sense to stereotype everyone who rides a motorcycle as a gang member, risk taker, and so forth. The more providers can avoid judging patients based on their behaviors and work to share information, power/control, and decision making the more effective the communication exchange will likely become.

Skills Exercise

In a conversation with a friend or loved one that lasts more than a couple of minutes, see whether you can focus on his or her eyes the entire time you and your friend are talking. Try to ignore the background, electronic devices, even an itch. When you're done, how did the experience feel—was it routine and the way you always talk with people? Or was it different for you and how did that difference impact your perception of the interaction? Ask the other person first whether he or she noticed anything different about the conversation? If he or she mentions the eye contact, ask how it made him or her feel about the conversation and about you as a friend/family member/lover?

Video Discussion Exercise

Analyze the video

- *Philadelphia* (1993)

Interactive Simulation Exercise

Pagano, M. (2015). *Communication case studies for health care professionals: An applied approach* (2nd ed.). New York, NY: Springer Publishing Company.

- Chapter 6, "Bad News" (pp. 55–66)
- Chapter 12, "I Understand" (pp. 123–132)
- Chapter 16, "I'm Feeling Better, But . . ." (pp. 161–172)

Health Care Issues in the Media

Health literacy and prescriptions
https://iom.nationalacademies.org/~/media/Files/Report%20Files/2004/Health-Literacy-A-Prescription-to-End-Confusion/healthliteracyfinal.pdf

How to improve doctor–patient communication
http://www.wsj.com/articles/SB10001424127887324050304578411251805908228

Health Communication Outcomes

As discussed in this and prior chapters, provider–patient communication is interpersonal and, in American culture, more often than not is based on both parties using narratives in order to share information. However, for providers who communicate using a biomedical, provider-centric, disease/injury-focused approach it is much more common to utilize closed-ended questioning as the way to gather patient information. Although this approach could make the interaction more focused and perhaps quicker than open-ended queries with a more narrative structure, the detective-like approach minimizes the opportunities for patient collaboration, trust building, shared decision making, and relationship development. In addition to the importance of providers using a more patient-centered communication style that encourages narratives and shared information, providers can nonverbally illustrate their interest in the patient vis-à-vis listening more than talking. By resisting the urge to dominate the conversation, providers can minimize the perception of themselves as paternalistic and authoritarian and instead nonverbally demonstrate their efforts to be collaborative and share both the power as well as the decision making in the relationship. Furthermore, providers need to carefully analyze their patients and use communication (verbal and nonverbal) behaviors that are appropriate based on the patient's demographics (age, sex, gender, education, literacy level, etc.). However, it is also essential that providers strive to avoid using stereotypes or treating patients differently based on their demographics, illness, behaviors, artifacts, and so forth. By resisting the urge to stereotype patients, providers have a much better opportunity to assimilate the information gathered in an unbiased manner and collaborate with patients regarding their health care decision making. Finally, the critical importance of recognizing the role literacy plays in effective interpersonal health communication cannot be overstated. Providers need to remind themselves that they speak a different language than their patients, using unique terminology. As a consequence, just as they would not try to communicate with an American-English speaker using an ethnic language the patient did not understand, the same logic applies to avoiding health care language/terminology with patients.

▪ REFERENCE

North Carolina State University. (2006). *Improving reading comprehension using metacognitive strategies: Fifth grade reading passages.* Retrieved from https://www.ncsu.edu/project/lancet/fifth_grade/hurricane5th.pdf

▪ BIBLIOGRAPHY

Deber, R., Kraetschmer, N., & Irvine, J. (1996). What role do patients wish to play in treatment decision-making? *Archives of Internal Medicine, 156,* 1414–1420.

Gawande, A. (2007). Better: A surgeon's notes on performance. In *Afterword: Suggestions for becoming a positive deviant* (pp. 249–257). New York, NY: Picador.

National Center for Education Statistics. (2015). *National assessment of adult literacy: Overview.* Retrieved from http://nces.ed.gov/naal/estimates/Overview.aspx

Osborne, H. (2013). *Health literacy from A to Z: Practical ways to communicate your health message* (2nd ed.). Burlington, MA: Jones & Bartlett.

Vernon, J., Trujillo, A., Rosenbaum, S., & DeBuono, B. (2007). *Low health literacy: Implications of national health policy.* Retrieved from http://sphhs.gwu.edu/departments/healthpolicy/CHPR/downloads/LowhealthLiteracyReport10_4_07.pdf

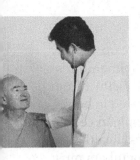

CHAPTER 5

Intercultural Communication in Health Care

For the purpose of this text, we are going to use the following as working definitions:

- *Acculturation:* the process of learning to be part of a new culture/coculture
- *Coculture:* a culture within a larger culture
- *Conflict:* differences in viewpoints; can be negative or positive
- *Culture:* the values, beliefs, rules, rituals, language, and behaviors of a group of people who share common goals
- *Diversity:* not just different cultures, but different perspectives
- *Intercultural communication:* information exchanges across cultures
- *Social identity:* how culture helps shape a person's identity

■ HEALTH CARE CULTURE—PROVIDERS

Perhaps you have not considered it previously, but health care can be viewed as a separate culture. It has its own set of values, rituals, and language. There are artifacts (clothing/uniforms) that are unique to the culture, there is a language that health care students must learn to be part of the culture, there are rituals: education, certification, licensing, continuing education, and so forth as well as values, most obviously, the Hippocratic Oath and caring for others. Think about how various cocultures in health care (MD/DO [doctor of osteopathy], RN, physician assistant [PA], etc.) have their own interdependent values, traditions, norms, and roles with the larger culture. And yet, in spite of role or philosophical differences for health care as a culture to produce positive outcomes and achieve its goals—the cocultures must work interdependently, using the same language to assure that patients receive the most effective care possible.

From a communication perspective, the culture of health care is truly unique. Members of the culture, regardless of their role or discipline/profession, are required to learn the language of health care, which is distinct from the participant's native language. This medical language is archived in books, taught in courses, and unique to the culture. And although people in certain industries use jargon to help their members adapt to their jobs, health care is one of the very few professions (law is another) in which members must learn an entire language separate from their native one, to become part of the heath care culture. Therefore, words like *appendicitis, aneurysm, selective serotonin reuptake inhibitor, lobectomy,* and so on are used to communicate anatomical, physiological, and observational realities. Health care as a culture can be evaluated based on its ability to adapt new members vis-à-vis educational programs such as medical, nursing, and physician assistant

Reflection 5.1. Why do many medical, nursing, and physician assistant programs have white-coat ceremonies for their students? How does this event help new members develop a sense of acculturation?

_____

_____

_____

_____

_____

schools. Although each of these cocultures teaches its students diverse perspectives on caring for ill and injured individuals as well as maintaining health, they do it using a common health care terminology/language; shared values and beliefs; and an appreciation for the ever-expanding interdisciplinary, interdependent nature of 21st-century health care delivery. As discussed in prior chapters, one of the distinctions between these cocultures centers around the pedagogical and philosophical approaches many nursing education programs take compared to programs for doctors and physician assistants. In the coculture of nursing, the biopsychosocial approach to health care is primarily the pedagogical focus. As compared to medical and physician assistant programs, where education tends to be more biomedical-centric. These cocultural differences have led to a more patient-focused, collaborative value and belief system for those who are nurses versus a more provider-centric, authoritarian approach, especially for doctors. However, as the culture of health care evolves, it appears that a patient-centric, collaborative approach may be gaining acceptance across cocultures. Clearly, that is one of the reasons for this text. However, as we explore the expanding role of intercultural communication (across cocultures and the larger U.S. culture), it is important to understand how the differences in cultures potentially impact provider–patient communication.

Reflection 5.2. Do you perceive the increasing efforts to have health care professionals work more collaboratively across cocultures/disciplines/professions as enhancing or detracting from intracultural and intercultural communication?

_____

_____

_____

_____

_____

Intercultural Communication—Patients and Families

One of the important realizations about health care is that patients and families are not part of the same culture as health care providers. Patients and families are part of the larger American culture, but not the health care culture. Again, for the most part, they do not share the language or have the same education, rituals, roles, beliefs, and behaviors. However, patients do share common goals with the providers who work with them—they all want the patient to be as healthy as possible. Therefore, the interpersonal communication and relationships we have been discussing can now be viewed in light of the intercultural nature of the health care context. In Chapter 4, health literacy was discussed; clearly health literacy is a direct result of the differences in non–health and health care cultures. If you go to a country where you are not a member of the culture, do not speak the language, know the beliefs, rituals, and so forth, you are likely going to feel isolated and insecure. In addition, because of the cultural differences, building trust is very difficult. Therefore, when health care providers recognize how patients can perceive their culture similar to an experience in a foreign culture, they can start to assess their communication—not just language—behaviors in terms of interacting interculturally. This recognition should encourage providers to strive to find ways to bridge the cultural differences to improve interpersonal and health communication and relationship development. As mentioned in Chapter 4, it is important to assess how much health care language a patient understands and can assimilate. Recognizing that behaviors necessary for the health care culture (haptics, proxemics, kinesics, data gathering, emotional restraint, etc.) may be antithetical to the larger patient culture, providers should be aware that common health care behaviors can make them appear uncaring, egocentric, and more focused on the disease than on the patient.

Part of the difference between the health care culture and the larger culture is that patients are accustomed to being the focus of attention when they pay for services. However, in health care, the focus is typically on the disease/injury and peripherally on the patient. In addition, legal issues specific to health care, such as medical records/patient privacy, malpractice risks, adverse events, treatment options, and so on, all impact provider–patient communication and can appear to patients as the provider being less concerned with them and more concerned with issues they do not know about (as nonmembers of the health care culture) and/or understand. Similarly, health care culture, unlike many other areas of the patient's culture, must be responsive to health insurers' requirements and, although the patient may want something different, the provider has little freedom to accommodate the patient based on the 21st-century health care culture's economic realities. All of these intercultural differences create communication problems for providers and patients and many of them are not even directly related to the illness/injury/health concerns that the provider–patient are addressing. However, the intra- and intercultural differences can impact both patients and providers.

Reflection 5.3. What if you have to tell a patient that there is a treatment for his or her illness, but the insurance company will not cover the cost and she or he cannot afford it? How do you suppose that information will impact the patient's perception of the health care culture generally, and you as a provider specifically? Understanding both sides of this issue from your health care culture perspective, how might you be able to enhance your provider–patient relationship?

_____

_____

_____

_____

_____

Social and Cultural Identities

One of the realities of acculturation is the likelihood that an individual's social and/or cultural identities will need to evolve. For example, part of membership in most health care cocultures, as well as the overall culture, is the recognition that providers will need to assume new identities. As medical, nursing, and physician assistant students become acculturated, they begin to understand that their new social/cultural identity will require them to behave differently, at least in the health care culture, than in the larger culture. For example, new members of the health care culture are cautioned against forming emotional attachments with their patients—as compared to other interpersonal relationships in the larger culture. As part of the health care culture, members are advised to seek patient disclosure of highly personal information but not to reciprocate, again distancing themselves from patients in spite of the need to form interpersonal relationships with them. Health care providers' roles may also require them to change their identities related to leadership, paternalistic, or even authoritarian communication behaviors depending on the context and the communication requirements.

Similarly, patients are frequently required to alter their identities based on the culture of health care and their illness or injury. Patients who previously were strong-willed, independent leaders may be forced to become dependent, exhausted, child-like followers of providers' orders. Or, based on the impact of the illness or injury, patients may undergo various identity responses (Charmaz, 1987):

- Supernormal: the patient does not want to let the illness or injury change himself or herself or their preillness/injury identity
- Restored: less optimistic about getting back to full preillness/injury self, but still won't believe there has been a change
- Contingent personal: recognizes he or she can no longer do what he or she used to and is starting to recognize changed identity
- Salvaged self: accepts new identity with some aspects of preillness/injury, coupled with current health realities

It is interesting to recognize that for the most part providers choose to become members of a culture and coculture that seeks to acculturate them by changing their social and cultural identities in part. However, patients generally have their identities impacted, often unwillingly, by the health care culture and/or in response to an illness or injury. Therefore, providers should recognize that many instances of patients' distrust, anger, hostility, and/or frustration may be the result of the impact of cultural differences and illness/injury as much as the specific health communication that appears to be the catalyst for patients' responses. The impact of changes in a patient's identity in health care culture versus the larger culture, as well as the shock of an illness/injury to a patient's sense of self may significantly contribute to problems in provider–patient communication, relationship development, and/or perceived outcomes. These social and cultural identity issues can be explored by examining verbal and nonverbal communication using an intercultural lens.

Reflection 5.4. How might a tumor or a cancer impact a patient's identity and how she or he communicates with a provider? How would you think the differences in culture between a patient and a provider might also be a potential issue?

Verbal and Nonverbal Intercultural Communication Issues

Expanding on the way intercultural communication potentially impacts provider–patient interactions, the differences in symbols/language create the most obvious problems. Most patients do not know or understand the language of health care and—just like when a person travels to a foreign country—many people in one culture do not stop to consider how people from another culture may be able to assimilate and/or understand their language. In health care, it is expected that providers will use health care terminology in their conversations about patients. However, providers must stop and analyze patients and/or patients' families and their knowledge of health care culture and language. Just as a person in Italy who speaks both Italian and English would need to determine whether someone from another culture could speak Italian and, if not, uses English in order to be understood, so must health care providers do with patients.

Clearly one way to determine whether patients understand the terms that providers are using is to ask patients to describe what they were told. Another way is to observe patients' nonverbal behaviors to see whether they are expressing confusion or a lack of comprehension. Providers must continually remind themselves that they speak two different languages in two distinct cultures; therefore, providers need to carefully assess the culture and literacy levels of patients, not just use health care language/terminology and assume patients understand. Similarly, providers need to be aware that the nonverbal cues associated with health care are very powerful. Whether it is the artifacts (white coats or scrub clothes), the edifices (hospitals, operating suites, MRI laboratories, etc.), or even the equipment (stethoscopes, examination tables, gloves, stirrups, etc.), these are unique to the health care culture and all remind the patient that she or he is not a member of the culture and thus not similar in many respects to those who are. Because of these dissimilarities, along with the language issues and other intercultural differences (e.g., health care providers are also using their cocultures/professions to earn a living), it should not be surprising to health care professionals or patients that there are communication issues vastly different from other interpersonal and/or professional-consumer aspects of their lives. Consequently, both providers and patients need to recognize the potential for intercultural conflict—both inter- and intraculturally.

Intercultural and Intracultural Conflict

As you know both as a consumer of health care (patient) and as a provider (or soon to be professional), the emotions, economics, and realities of health care delivery affect every aspect of the provider–patient relationship. These various realities can lead to both intercultural (provider and patient) and provider–provider (intracultural) conflict. Although the obvious distinctions from language issues, especially patients who do not speak/understand American English, is the most apparent risk to effective interpersonal and health communication, there are numerous other culturally related potential problems for communicators.

As one of the biggest budget areas in the American economy, the impact of health care delivery and services creates not only hardships, but nearly unimaginable decisions for some patients. And although some of these economic conflicts are easily recognizable for providers (e.g., prescriptions that cost tens of thousands of dollars per year, procedures that are not covered by health insurance), some may not be unless the provider specifically seeks the information needed to assess them.

 Research Exercise 5a. Let's do a little health care economics research. Use the Internet or phone a health care facility (provider office, hospital, pharmacy, insurer, etc.) and find the price of two prescription medications (cash price versus price with your insurance; not the copay but the overall charge) Zithromax (single pills or Z-pack) and Crestor, 10 mg (30 tablets) in your city. Get the prices at two or three very different-style local pharmacies (e.g., CVS versus Costco). Next, look for the national average cost for a single coronary artery stent (total charges, hospital, and physician) procedure with all the needed diagnostic tests and so forth to see whether you can find out what your insurance would pay for this procedure and what your copay would be. Finally, discuss these costs and how they might impact provider–patient communication differently based on a patient having health insurance versus a patient who is uninsured.

As mentioned previously, unless a provider seeks more information it may not be obvious whether the patient is living alone, with family, in a shelter, or on the street. Similarly, without assessment and inquiry, it may not be at all clear whether she or he can afford even modestly priced prescriptions. And the realities of the current American health care system which is clearly economically tiered, may also present severe conflict issues for many patients. Therefore, it is important for providers to frequently remind themselves about how economics affect access to health care in America (see Figure 5.1).

Clearly, the realities of Figure 5.1 for American health care providers and patients are both troubling and critically important to understand. As the pyramid illustrates, for the wealthiest U.S. citizens any health care is possible, from plastic surgery to concierge medicine (a provider who is on a retainer and available for telephone, electronic, or home visits 24/7/365). However, for the overwhelming majority of Americans, this level of health care and its options (access to the most prestigious hospitals and specialists, diagnostic tests, and treatments) are unavailable. For most patients in this country, health care access is based on private

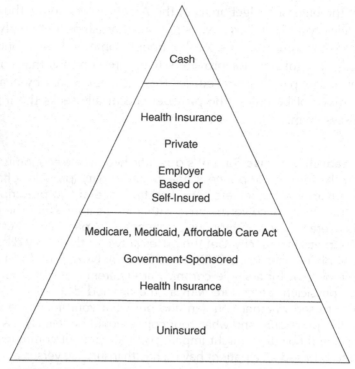

FIGURE 5.1. Tiered U.S. Health Care Access

(employer-based or self-insured) health insurance and whether or not they can see a certain provider, have a procedure performed, tests paid for, and so on based on their policy and the amount of copay the insurance requires the patient to contribute to the cost of office/hospital visits, medications, diagnostic tests, and so forth. Therefore, although these patients have less access than those who can pay cash for any type of health care access/delivery, the insured have a number of choices regarding their providers, hospitals, and services. For patients who must rely on government-sponsored health care plans (often administered by private firms but paid in part by the federal and/or state governments), their options for health care access are markedly reduced compared to the top two tiers. Patients in the third tier of the pyramid in Figure 5.1 can generally only see providers who accept government-sponsored health insurance programs. Consequently, many patients who are on Medicare and Medicaid especially are very limited in which providers will accept their insurance. Finally, the 30-plus million Americans who are uninsured in this country have very limited access to health care. Most providers will not see patients who do not have insurance and/or cash to pay for services. Similarly, many diagnostic (not life-threatening emergency procedures/tests) procedures and treatments are unattainable for those in the bottom tier of the pyramid. Consequently, the uninsured typically are forced to use the emergency department (ED) for their health care, regardless of whether it is a toothache or a sore throat. There are very few community-type centers available (from transportation, hours of operation, geographic perspectives, etc.) to the uninsured in major cities and far fewer, if any, in small-town and rural America.

Reflection 5.5. What issues from health communication, information exchange, and intercultural communication perspectives do you see as related to tiered access to U.S. health care delivery from both provider and patient viewpoints?

_____

_____

_____

_____

_____

The issues related to health care economics and patient access in this country clearly create communication and relationship development problems for patients and providers. However, in addition to the intercultural problems discussed previously, there are also intracultural conflicts that impact health communication, provider–provider relationships, and health care delivery.

Chapter 10 focuses specifically on provider–provider communication; however, because of the cultural issues related to cocultures in health care working interdependently to accomplish common—patient, organization, and individual—goals, it is important to address the intracultural aspects of health care delivery. As mentioned previously, among the potential intracultural issues in communicating across disciplines/professions are the differences in philosophical approaches, but also the changing organizational approach, from single leader (physician) to a team (doctor, nurse, PA, advanced practice registered nurse [APRN], etc.) perspective, which increases the need for effective provider–provider communication across cocultures. And it requires members of the health care culture, regardless of the coculture, to try to find the most appropriate approach to patient care based on the individual patient, but also the patient's collaboration and participation in decision making. The potential conflict among providers, especially those from different cocultures, must be recognized and assessed to minimize any potential distractions. Also, within cocultures (e.g., physicians), there can be conflict across disciplines as when the patient's primary care provider and cardiologist disagree on the diagnosis or the most appropriate treatment plan. Similarly, nursing staff could have a conflict with a nursing supervisor who felt that more time should be spent on documentation than on patient interaction. The intracultural conflicts within the health care culture and/or within health care cocultures need to be recognized by providers—assessed and addressed. Therefore, it is vitally important for providers to recognize the potential communication problems that could lead to untoward diagnostic, treatment, and/or wellness outcomes. However, the barriers to effective health and interpersonal/intercultural communication also contribute to the potential for intercultural conflict.

Intercultural Barriers to Health Communication

Unfortunately, there are a number of intercultural barriers to effective health communication, including:

- Patients and providers who do not use American English as their primary language

- Providers who do not understand or address the issues related to communication with patients who are not members of the health care culture

- Patients whose economic situation negatively impacts their access to care and/or treatments

- Perceived differences in socioeconomic status (SES) between patients and providers

Reflection 5.6. Based on the discussions in this chapter and prior chapters, what are some communication strategies that can overcome some of the barriers to effective intercultural health communication between providers and patients?

_____

_____

_____

_____

_____

It should not be surprising that patients who are not native American-English speakers will have difficulty assimilating, assessing, and utilizing health communication that is not appropriate for their literacy level. However, it is important to also recognize that it may be just as difficult for patients whose first language is American English if they are communicating with a provider who does not use American English as his or her first language. Consequently, providers must also assess their language usage, especially if they are not native speakers. As mentioned earlier, sharing symbols/language is critically important to attaining interpersonal/health communication goals and developing/building interpersonal relationships. It should not be surprising that regardless of whether a communicator is a patient or a provider, intercultural language barriers create enormous problems for all interactants and need to be addressed—vis-à-vis a translator or appropriate literacy level—in order for providers and patients to have the best chance for effective health communication information exchange and decision making.

Similarly, the disparities between the larger culture and the health care culture and cocultures need to be recognized by providers as potential barriers to effective interpersonal health communication. Providers need to assess whether patients not only understand the health care language that is being used, but the various diagnostic issues and treatment options available—including the differences in roles and responsibilities for various providers/cocultures (specialists, allied health professionals, etc.). It is not uncommon, for example, for some patients to not understand the differences in roles and responsibilities for APRNs and PAs versus MD/DOs and/or RNs. Clarifying who is caring for them, the provider's role, educational background, supervision, and so on can make it much easier for patients to trust all members of the health care team and feel safe sharing information and collaborating with various members of the health care culture and coculture.

One of the most difficult intercultural barriers is related to economic issues in U.S. health care. Within the U.S. culture, there are various cocultures related to health care access, as illustrated in Figure 5.1. However, this lack of access creates numerous barriers related to both communication and clinical issues. The increased wait in EDs in this country related to uninsured patients, need for chronic care in an acute care setting creates frustration and problems for both health care providers and patients (with insurance and without insurance). Because it is illegal to refuse to see a patient in the ED, everyone who wants to be seen must be examined. Consequently, many EDs have 2- to 3-hour wait times for admission to the ED and everyone—patients and providers—find this a very perplexing situation. Providers generally choose the ED coculture because they want to take care of urgent and/or acute care problems, but are faced with increasing numbers of patients who have nowhere else to go for their chronic or nonacute health care. And patients, whether they have insurance or not, are having to wait and then, because of the prolonged wait times and numbers of patients to be seen, often do not get as much time with the ED provider as they perceive they should—which further impacts their frustration as well as their information exchange, collaborations in decision making, and/or relationship building/trust. Finally, the cost of health care treatments especially can be extremely problematic for patients who need a drug or procedure, but also for providers who want to help patients but have little or no control over the cost of care or what is approved/paid for by insurers. Thus, the economic barriers to effective intercultural provider–patient communication are both pervasive and frustrating for patients and providers alike.

In addition, as discussed in Chapter 4, the differences in SES between providers and many patients also contribute to the problems in effective intercultural health communication. The inability of patients to perceive any similarity with providers who are clearly in different economic, social, educational, and professional contexts makes it less likely for patients to want to develop an interpersonal relationship or cross-cultural trust. Just as with the other barriers to effective intercultural health communication, providers need to realize these potential issues and attempt to address them with patients and overcome them if wellness and/or illness goals are to be attained.

Reflections (among the possible responses)

5.1. Why do many medical, nursing, and physician assistant programs have white-coat ceremonies for their students? How does this event help new members develop a sense of acculturation?

Among the major hallmarks of a culture are the language and traditions that differentiate it from other cultures. In the health care culture, there is a distinctive language/medical terminology used by its members. However, health care also uses unique artifacts to differentiate itself from other cultures—white coats and scrub suits are two of the most obvious artifacts that identify health care providers. In fact, it is rare for a patient to ever question a provider's credibility/education during an initial interaction; a primary reason for this unusual behavior is that in the larger U.S. culture, the artifacts and contexts (offices, hospitals, etc.) provide the nonverbal assurances for patients that whoever is wearing a white coat and/or scrub clothes is presumed to be a health care provider and no other documentation is required. Therefore, the act of conferring a white coat or a labeled scrub suit on a new member of a culture is part of the acculturation process and helps that student (MD/DO, RN, PA, etc.) adapt to his or her new role, responsibilities, and membership.

5.2. Do you perceive the increasing efforts to have health care professionals work more collaboratively across cocultures/disciplines/professions as enhancing or detracting from intracultural and intercultural communication?

As cocultures collaborate, instead of viewing their roles from a hierarchical perspective, the opportunities for expanding input, information sharing, diverse viewpoints, and enhanced outcomes for both providers and patients become more possible. Working in teams, where all members have not only interdependent roles and responsibilities but also the potential to impact group decision making and institutional as well as patient-centered goals, has the potential to enhance intercultural (across cocultures) communication. For patients and providers, greater collaboration across health care cocultures (specialists, disciplines, professions) offers the opportunity to increase information exchanges, decrease monologues/authoritarian behaviors, enhance relationship development, and improve common goal attainment for all.

5.3. What if you have to tell a patient that there is a treatment for his or her illness but the insurance company will not cover the cost and he or she cannot afford it? How do you suppose that information will impact the patient's perception of the health care culture generally, and you as a provider specifically? Understanding both sides of this issue from your health care culture perspective, how might you be able to enhance your provider–patient relationship?

One of the most difficult situations a provider can face is having to relate the economic realities of health care to a patient who either does not have the insurance or financial ability to cover the costs of necessary treatment options. It would not be surprising for a patient and/or family members in this situation to blame the provider or the health care culture. Although these arguments may have some merit they will not help your patient's condition or outcome. The patient's and family members' frustrations and anger are understandable, but the provider needs to try to help them move beyond the initial responses and find other potential options for care. For example, perhaps the provider could contact a pharmaceutical representative or a pharmaceutical company to see whether there is a prescription assistance program for which the patient might qualify. Or suggest the family contact a local, regional, or national nonprofit association that might have some funding options (e.g., American Heart Association, Susan G. Komen breast cancer fund). Furthermore, the provider can use empathic listening to show support for the patient's anger and frustration but also to illustrate the provider's willingness to try and help the patient as much as possible. Often, patients appreciate provider's efforts, even if they are ultimately unsuccessful, to help them overcome a clinical or nonclinical problem because it demonstrates the provider's caring and willingness to be more than a member of the health care culture.

5.4. How might a tumor or a cancer impact a patient's identity and how she or he communicates with a provider? How would you think the differences in culture between a patient and a provider might also be a potential issue?

As discussed in this and prior chapters, communication does not take place in a vacuum. Interpersonal communication is dependent on context, communicator, and culturally dependent. Therefore, as the context for a patient's health/wellness evolves, the patient's communication with the provider may be directly impacted. The patient may become more withdrawn (in denial), angry, or resentful. However, the provider needs to understand these responses are related to the patient's sense of self-identity and how the illness/injury impacts the patient's self-perceptions. Similarly, the differences in the cultures of patients and providers may also play a role in how the patient chooses to communicate. For example, if the patient perceives the provider, a member of the health care culture, as emotionally detached, uncaring, or operating from a biomedical approach, the patient may feel that his or her concerns will not be important to the provider. Similarly, the patient may question whether the provider's ability to make money off of the patient's illness/injury is the major focus for the provider's role in their relationship. Therefore, it is important for the provider to understand how the communication context is markedly changed by a patient's illness or injury and to be even more attuned to the patient's verbal and nonverbal behaviors. The differences in cultures related to illness/injury—especially the routinizing of serious, even terminal illnesses and injuries for members of the health care culture—must be perceived as antithetical to the experiences/expectations of most patients in the larger U.S. culture. Therefore, every effort should be made by providers in such contexts to communicate in a more interpersonal and empathic style.

5.5. What issues from health communication, information exchange, and intercultural communication perspectives do you see as related to tiered access to U.S. health care delivery from both provider and patient viewpoints?

The tiered U.S. health care system creates enormous communication problems for providers and patients alike. Except for the wealthiest Americans, everyone else in this country is striving to understand his or her access realities. Even those with private health insurance likely do not know the ramifications of their policies' limitations in terms of provider access, diagnostic tests, and/or treatments. In consequence, these issues become part of the provider–patient conversation and impact provider and/or patient decision making. And certainly, for patients who have government-based health insurance or no insurance, their communication with providers is further obfuscated and/or minimized by the limited access they have to care based on their insurance policies' requirements or the lack of insurance. Similarly, providers may be placed in the difficult position of knowing of a treatment option but trying to decide whether it should be discussed with the patient knowing that it would be cost prohibitive.

5.6. Based on the discussions in this chapter and prior chapters, what are some communication strategies that can overcome some of the barriers to effective intercultural health communication between providers and patients?

Although there are numerous barriers to effective intercultural health communication between patients and providers, most of them can be decreased through active listening, appropriate language choices, interpersonal communication, and interpersonal relationship building. Although there are many distinctions among the health care culture and its cocultures and the larger U.S. culture, providers who are willing to understand these differences and work to overcome them can clearly help diminish many of the barriers. For example, the use of professional translators with patients who are not fluent in American English is one step in improving health communication across cultures. Another is the assessment of a patient's health literacy level and the level-appropriate intercultural health communication/education. Furthermore, recognizing the issues created by SES differences between providers and patients as well as the economic obstacles created by U.S. tiered health care access—affords providers an opportunity to address these potential problems openly with patients using empathic listening and critical thinking to try to help patients as much as possible.

Skills Exercise

Try to have a conversation with someone who speaks a language that you do not understand. How frustrating is that for you? Was it also difficult for the other person? How might this frustration impact your perception of the other person and/or him or her of you? Now what if your prescription label looked like this to you, "afjafj ladfjdaf;ajfdal;jfdl;k afdafjf; afjdf a day?" How would you know what to do with the medication—whether to swallow or chew it? When to take it? How often? What were its side effects? How might a provider help a patient overcome these literacy/language obstacles?

Video Discussion Exercise

Analyze the video

■ *Patch Adams* (1998)

Interactive Simulation Exercise

Pagano, M. (2015). *Communication case studies for health care professionals: An applied approach* (2nd ed.). New York, NY: Springer Publishing Company.

■ Chapter 37, "No Hablo Español" (pp. 357–366)

■ Chapter 40, "Please Take Off Your Clothes and Put on This Gown" (pp. 383–390)

■ Chapter 44, "Why Am I Not Seeing a Doctor?" (pp. 415–422)

Health Care Issues in the Media

Health literacy
https://iom.nationalacademies.org/~/media/Files/Report%20Files/2004/Health-Literacy-A-Prescription-to-End-Confusion/healthliteracyfinal.pdf

Prescription labels
http://www.nytimes.com/2005/10/25/health/policy/and-now-a-warning-about-labels.html

Health Communication Outcomes

As Americans we are members of larger cultures, the world, but also numerous cocultures: Italian, French, Hispanic, your family, school, professional organization, and so on. One of the nonnational/nonethnic cultures is health care. This unique culture is different from American culture in that the health culture has its own distinct language/terminology, values, beliefs, and goals. It has culture-specific artifacts, roles, and traditions. However, the differences in the larger U.S. and health care cultures often contribute to the verbal and nonverbal communication problems that can negatively impact provider–patient interactions. As providers try to manipulate the differences between these cultures, they often fail to recognize the importance of sharing symbols/language as well as social and cultural identities. Because of differences in culture and SES, there are frequently barriers to effective information exchange, trust building, and collaborative communication and decision making. These barriers contribute to potential intercultural conflict and further create provider–patient health communication difficulties.

■ REFERENCE

Charmaz, K. (1987). Struggling for a self: Identity level of the chronically ill. In J. Roth & P. Conrad (Eds.), *Research in the sociology of health care* (pp. 283–321). Greenwich, CT: JAI Press.

■ BIBLIOGRAPHY

Ford, L., & Yep, G. (2003). Working along the margins: Developing community-based strategies for communicating about health with marginalized groups. In T. Thompson, A. Dorsey, K. Miller, & R. Parrott (Eds.), *Handbook of health communication* (pp. 241–261). Mahwah, NJ: Erlbaum.

Gawande, A. (2007). *Better: A surgeon's notes on performance, "Naked"* (pp. 73–83). New York, NY: Picador.

Kreps, G. (2006). Communication and racial inequalities in health care. *American Behavioral Scientist, 49,* 1–15.

Sharif, I., Lo, S., & Ozuah, P. (2006). Availability of Spanish prescription labels. *Journal of Health Care for the Poor and Underserved, 17*(1), 67.

Smedley, B., Stith, A., & Nelson, A. (Eds.). (2003). *Unequal treatment: Confronting racial and ethnic disparities in health care.* Retrieved from http://www.nap.edu/catalog/12875.html

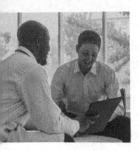

CHAPTER 6

Ethics and Health Care

For the purpose of this text, we are going to use the following as working definitions:

- *Autonomy:* Ability to make unilateral decisions, especially about topics in which you have expertise

- *Conflict of interest:* Making decisions or offering services that provide one person/organization with a financial advantage over another option/alternative

- *Health Insurance Portability and Accountability Act (HIPAA):* Federal legislation that controls patients' access to care and the privacy of their medical information

- *Informed consent:* Providing patients with sufficient information, in a manner they can understand and assimilate, so they can agree or disagree to a planned procedure, treatment, or strategy

- *Shared decision making:* A patient's right to partner with a provider in the patient's health care decisions

- *Theory of justice:* Fairness; people receiving what is rightly theirs

- *Theory of rights:* Claims a person can make on a culture or individuals

- *Utilitarian theory:* The benefits of an action outweigh the harm, or making decisions based on the greater good

■ AUTONOMY

As previously discussed, for health care providers, autonomy covers multiple areas. First, over the centuries, *autonomy* in health care has frequently referred to providers', principally physicians', authority to make decisions for and/or with patients regarding their diagnoses and treatments. Over the past two decades there has been an effort to increase patients' roles in collaborating with providers, which could be seen as limiting the provider's autonomy. However, the larger issue regarding autonomy in the past three decades is related to the provider's ability to make decisions alone, or in partnership with the patient, about diagnostic tests, treatments, and/or procedures. This decrease in autonomy will be further discussed in Chapter 7, but is related to the impact of insurers and their managed care demands.

From an ethical perspective, not an economic one, autonomy necessarily presents several key health communication questions for both providers and patients:

1. Who should be making health care decisions for mentally competent adults?

2. How does the patient's health knowledge impact his or her right to make health care decisions?

3. What are potential consequences for provider autonomy in patient decision making?

Because there are laws in every state to govern health care decision making for children and mentally incompetent adults, this discussion is only related to mentally competent 18-year-old and older patients.

Reflection 6.1. After all your education, clinical training, and health care experience, who do you think is most capable of making decisions about a patient's care, you or the patient? Why?

_____

_____

_____

_____

_____

From an ethical perspective providers must decide how much information to share with patients, what role the provider intends to play in the decision making, and how or how much to include the patient in his or her illness/injury/ wellness care plan. It is very likely that you can feel the dialectical tensions in these issues: (a) as a patient you likely want to be constantly involved in decision making—as a provider, you can envision the potential time, costs, and problems that can arise from collaborative decision making; (b) as a provider you recognize the differences in your knowledge, expertise, and skills compared to a patient. However, you also realize that if you are wrong, you are solely responsible for the outcomes and that creates potential relational, moral, and legal issues.

These dialectical tensions are illustrative of the ethical dilemmas providers face on a regular basis. Although it is true that providers have more knowledge and experience than almost all of their potential patients—it is ultimately the patient's life that is being impacted by the decision making. Similarly, it is widely accepted that one of the key health care provider roles is to educate patients about their health, illness, and/or injury. Therefore, even with the differences in education and experience/expertise, ethically, patients should have a right to make decisions about what happens to them. Clearly, there are emergency conditions in which this may not be possible, but apart from those, providers need to use effective health and interpersonal communication to educate and empower patients and encourage them to collaborate in the decision making. Although this power sharing and participative approach may not alleviate all of the provider's legal and ethical obligations, it will offer him or her the opportunity to work with the patient as a partner rather than an authority figure who is making unilateral decisions. Consequently, to avoid using autonomy as a demonstration of power and control, providers can use effective health and interpersonal communication to educate, build trust and relationships, and make shared assessments.

As with most decisions in 21st-century America, when customers/clients are less knowledgeable than the service provider (e.g., auto repair, computer viruses/software, and retirement plans), they expect to be informed in a language/terminology he or she can understand and assimilate, given an opportunity to answer questions, and, if desired, get a second (or third) opinion. Therefore, providers need to not only recognize these expectations from U.S. culture, but use them as a way to enhance their provider–patient relationship and minimize or eliminate ethical concerns regarding decision making. Before ordering nonemergent tests, procedures, and/or treatments, providers should ask themselves, "Have I explained to the patient what I think is best and why?" Such internal assessments by the provider allows for interpersonal communication with the patient that includes appropriate educational information sharing, as well as the provider's reasoning for the particular studies, medications, and/or surgery. By assuring that the patient is not only aware of what is planned, but educated and agrees to it minimizes unethical risks and/or autonomous behaviors. However, sharing control of decision making with patients is only as ethical as the honesty, literacy-appropriateness, and completeness of the information provided.

■ TRUTH TELLING

Although it is true that patients expect to be informed about their illness/injury/wellness plans, it is also true that they expect such information to be factual and complete. All too often providers must decide not just whether to provide information to patients, but how much and in what manner. For example, when a terminally ill patient asks if a treatment option is really viable, it is not uncommon for some providers to exaggerate the potential for such a treatment for that particular patient, "of course, there's always a chance that this will work when others did not." Although it is true that nothing is impossible, providers must constantly ask themselves whether they are providing truthful information that patients can use to make decisions. In the previous example, if the provider has answered completely and honestly, "it is very unlikely that it will work in your case. We can try it, but it may make you feel worse and you might not get to enjoy your time with your family as much" the patient has more accurate information to base his or her decision on. It is often difficult to discuss death and dying with patients and families, but to use false hope as a way to avoid educating the patient/family about the realities of the situation, risks further shortening the patient's quality of life and time to address other issues (e.g., family, insurance, finances, and friends). Remembering that the biomedical model is about fixing a problem, those who seek to communicate using such an approach are likely going to have great difficulty admitting first to themselves and then to their patients when an illness/injury cannot be fixed. As a consequence, to continue to find a "fix," providers may give patients false hope or continue futile treatments, both of which only serve to diminish the patient's quality of life and minimize her or his truth-filled decision-making opportunities (e.g., see videos, *Miss Evers' Boys* [1997] and/or *Wit* [2001]). Although autonomy and truth telling raise serious ethical questions for health care providers, maintaining patient confidentiality is also a critical issue.

Reflection 6.2. You have a young female patient with a large abdominal mass and the patient wants to know whether the tumor/surgery will keep her from getting pregnant. The scans and tests suggest that the tumor will likely require the removal of at least one ovary and tube, but could require a total hysterectomy and it could be a cancerous tumor, but you will not know until you operate. How will you answer her preoperation question and why?

_____

_____

_____

_____

_____

■ CONFIDENTIALITY

Patients have the right to expect providers to keep their health information confidential and not share it with anyone without permission. In addition, there are laws to protect patient's rights in this area that will be discussed in Chapter 12. However, providers are expected, both ethically and legally, to protect individual patient's identities, diagnoses, hospitalizations, and so forth. These expectations are often challenged by information requests from employers, insurers, family, friends, and/or the media. Therefore, it is imperative when providers are communicating with patients that both parties recognize the desire for confidentiality and the realities of 21st-century health care. Specifically, patients need to be knowledgeable, understanding that the provider will share all patient information with the health insurer and sign a consent form that makes this fact clear if they intend to use health care insurance for their payments. If the patient refuses, then the provider cannot share the patient record and the patient will be responsible for paying all of his or her bill (this is also true for hospital and/or other health care organization services). Similarly, if patients have work-related injuries, and want to have their health care bills paid for by workers' compensation insurance, then patients need to consent to having their health care information available to both their employer and the workers' compensation insurer. For the most part, these confidentiality issues are governed by the patient's willingness to share health information with insurers (and employers in the case of workers' compensation), or to individually pay for services himself or herself. However, it is imperative for providers and health care organizations to make sure that patients understand what they are agreeing to when they sign the consent-to-release-information forms.

Therefore, it is important for providers to verify that patients are informed and have signed the appropriate consent-to-release-information forms before the provider communicates with anyone—insurer, employer, or others. However, in today's health care environment, one of the most important aspects of confidentiality relates to HIPAA, passed by Congress and signed into law in 1996. HIPAA requires health care organizations and providers to protect patients' confidentialities (except for workers' compensation) as directed by the patient. Therefore, not only can patients determine whether health insurance companies can have access to their health information, but also patients must decide what if any data about an illness/injury the patient's family, friends, or anyone can be told.

Reflection 6.3. You are working in an emergency department (ED) and a woman who says she is the mother of a 20-year-old patient being treated for alcohol intoxication calls to inquire whether her daughter is in your facility. What do you tell her or do, and why?

_____

_____

_____

_____

_____

Although confidentiality is a very important part of modern health care delivery and health communication it does create several ethical issues for providers. For example, in Reflection 6.3, does your answer change if the patient is too mentally impaired to make a decision? What if the woman on the phone says she needs to catch a plane to come to take care of the

patient—if she's in your emergency department (ED)? But sometimes confidentiality becomes an ethical issue because providers want to share information about a patient/experience with friends.

You are helping deliver twins and you decide, without any permission, it
would be great to share the birth (with a picture of babies and mom in the background) on Facebook—is this unethical, or a breach of patient confidentiality?
The answer is yes; health care providers have no right to share patient's photos, or any health-related information without the patient's written permission
and based on your organization's policies. Similarly, you are in the ED and a
celebrity is a patient, not only is it a breach of HIPAA and confidentiality to
post on social media the person's name, but it is just as unethical and also
a HIPAA violation if you tell your parents or spouse that the celebrity was a
patient there—even if you do not disclose the patient's illness/injury/reason
for treatment. Providers need to constantly remind themselves that they need
to treat any and all patient information as confidential unless the patient has
specifically given written permission for its release. The best rule for communicating patient information is to be sure the patient has approved it first, if not,
get permission, or do not discuss it with anyone. Although it is both an ethical and a legal requirement to get patients' permission to release their health
information—consent for care is another critically important communication
issue for health providers to understand and adhere to.

■ CONSENT FOR CARE

Consent for care (also known as informed consent) is both a legal and an
ethical issue. The legal aspects related to consent for care will be discussed in
Chapter 13. However, from a health communication perspective it is important to recognize the provider's role in educating patients in obtaining their
consent for care (see Skloot, 2010). The critically important reality for providers
is the ethical need to assure that the patient understands the specifics of the
planned procedure that he or she is consenting to, any alternate possibilities,
as well as potential adverse events and their probabilities. As you can surmise,
this interpersonal communication requires a provider to insure that his or her
views of autonomy and truth telling do not conflict with both the ethical and
legal intent of informed consent requirements.

The goal of educating patients about procedures, treatments, and/or services
is to help them make accurately informed decisions. Consequently, providers
need to carefully use language (verbally and written) that the patient understands and assimilates, but also provide ample time to address questions and/or
concerns. Providers should rely on their verbal and nonverbal communication
to not only provide information, but seek feedback to determine the patient's
level of understanding, confusion, or misperceptions. Although it is important
to educate the patient prior to signing consent forms, do you think you have
any responsibility to educate yourself about the costs of health care services/
treatments/plans that you might recommend and/or order for your patients?

Reflection 6.4. Have you been asked to sign a consent form for a procedure/ test/service? If so, did you feel fully informed? If not, why not? And if not, did you feel comfortable asking the provider for more information or clarification?

_____

_____

_____

_____

_____

■ PAYING FOR HEALTH CARE

There are various types of ethical issues related to patient's rights and justice; however, one aspect of health care ethics that is less frequently discussed from a provider perspective is the cost of health care and its impact on provider–patient interactions, decision making, and outcomes. Although it may be true that health care providers can only control certain aspects of health care costs (if in private practice) and then primarily if they accept health insurance they will be paid what is the agreed upon rate with the insurer. However, because the costs of health care visits, procedures, and hospitalization are obfuscated, if available, for patients— based on insurance policies and the diagnosis-related group (DRG) payment system for providers and organizations—and the cost of medications and ther- apies are often unknown even by the providers who order them or deliver the services, the question of ethics related to information sharing seems appropriate.

If you are going to recommend a procedure or a medication to a patient, doesn't the patient have the right to know what the cost of that decision will be (copay, deductible, out-of-pocket, etc.)? Do you feel the health care provider has a role in assessing treatment decisions with patients that include cost dis- cussions? For example, if you feel that a Z-pack (Azithromycin) will be the best antibiotic because it requires only 5 versus 10 days of treatment. However, it will cost the patient $90 versus $10 for amoxicillin; shouldn't that information be part of the decision-making collaboration between you and the patient? Clearly, in order to provide this type of data you may need help from the phar- maceutical representatives for the various products you prescribe.

From an ethical perspective, at what point is the cost of health care as important as the diagnosis, treatment possibilities, and so forth? Does it make any sense to order blood pressure medications, diabetes treatments, and cholesterol-lowering medicines for a 70-year-old if that patient cannot afford to buy them? However, if the provider is not discussing the costs of these treatments along with the rest of the information being shared with the patient, how can either the provider or the patient make an informed decision? And how ethical is it for the patient to arrive at the pharmacy expecting to get medications only to find out that the copays and/or deductibles make it impossible for him or her to purchase the therapies? At that point, the patient is communicating with a pharmacist who does not know the patient's health history or socioeconomic status, and consequently can only focus on what the insurance company will pay for the prescribed treatment and how much the patient needs to pay. The patient then must either ask the pharmacist to communicate the problem to the provider and try to find an alternative plan, or try to contact the provider himself or herself to discuss a solution. However, it is likely that the provider will not be able to talk when the patient calls, so the patient will need to either wait at the pharmacy or leave and return later when/if an economic and pharmacologic solution can be found.

As we continue to seek a more patient-centric approach to health care, shouldn't the cost of procedures and therapies be available to both providers and patients? From an ethical perspective—keeping in mind the need to share health information—isn't that information critical if a truly informed decision is to be made? For many elderly in the United States living on a fixed income, if they are to have sufficient food and shelter there is only so much money available for health care costs. And although it can be argued that no one should have to decide between food and prescriptions, it is also true that providers are generally not the arbiters of most health care charges. Nonetheless, the realities are the same, patients and providers can only make empowered decisions if the costs of one option versus another are part of the discussion. Think about other areas of your life, you need to have the plumbing fixed in your bathroom, do you not get an estimate on what that will cost before you make a decision on how to proceed? The same is true of almost every other consumer purchase in American culture. We don't go pick out a shirt at a store and wait until we get to the register to find out that it is too expensive for our budget. And yet in health care, one of the major cost drivers in our economy, this is what happens to patients all the time. They are recommended treatments, procedures, services and not told for the most part what they will cost until they complete the selection (point of sale) or even afterward when they receive a notice from the insurer that the patients' bills exceeded their insurance benefits.

Reflection 6.5. How would you respond if you went to a store and nothing you needed had a price on it? So every time you went to buy something, you could not determine whether you could afford it until you were ready to check out. What are the parallels to patient's experiences with tests/procedures/treatment costs and the lack of pricing/billing information prior to a patient's decision making?

_____

_____

_____

_____

_____

The ethical implications of health care costs and provider–patient communication are seldom discussed, but providers need to consider how ethical it is to make recommendations for things that they either do not know the cost of (from the particular patient's perspective) or they do not want to take the time to learn what the patient can afford and what the best options are to meet the patient's health and economic needs. As you likely recognize, this brings the discussion back to the biopsychosocial approach to health care delivery. If a provider is using communication to learn about the patient's biological, psychological, and sociological history, then the provider will have information already gathered about the patient's economic situation (working full or part time, retired, on a pension, homeless, etc.). However, if the provider is focusing only on the disease/injury, then the diagnosis and treatment (apart from the patient's ability to pay for it) are the critical elements for the provider and the ethics of affordable options are not part of the provider's communication equation. Consequently, in consideration of ethics and effective information sharing, and collaborative decision making, striving to help patients understand the full implications (including costs) of their diagnosis and treatment options should be a critical part of providers' health and interpersonal communication. Such an approach should help to avoid unethical treatment/services/procedure recommendations that impact a patient's quality of life and/or death.

■ QUALITY OF LIFE AND/OR DEATH

As you explore the many ethical issues related to provider–patient communication, perhaps none is more troubling than those related to a patient's quality of life and/or death. Health care providers, especially those working with a biomedical approach, often continue to confront illnesses and/or injuries with rigor and vigor even when patients are confronting terminal outcomes. Consequently, from an ethical perspective, the question arises: At what point should the patient be informed of the realities of the situation, along with the risks, realistic advantages versus disadvantages of various plans, and so on?

Although Chapter 14 discusses end-of-life communication in more detail, here we are exploring discussions of quality of life/death with an ethical lens. Clearly, we could reiterate the ethical issues related to the costs of fighting death regardless of the patient's realities, but instead let us focus on trying to navigate the dialectical tension between curing a disease and providing the best quality of life possible. Obviously, providers cannot predict the future; however, it is often obvious when a patient has reached a state at which further aggressive treatment is unlikely to offer any positive outcomes and may in fact cause added pain, discomfort, and/or limited ability for interpersonal communication with friends, family, and/or a significant other. Providers need to use their intrapersonal communication to assess whether they are attempting to offer the patient the best quality of life/death possible, or whether they are trying to battle death (failure from a biomedical perspective) at any cost (to patient, family, and/or economic) in order to fulfill their own self-worth values, and/or beliefs. Knowledgeable, experienced providers always assess the potential benefits and outcomes for any treatment plan. However, when the provider uses autonomy and does not educate and collaborate with a patient/family about a patient's treatment (or lack thereof) decision making, the patient is clearly not being given his or her right to make informed choices about various treatment plans.

Reflection 6.6. You are an ED provider treating a patient who has stage IV cancer and has not responded to surgery, chemotherapy, or radiation. The patient has a living will and advance directive that clearly state her desire not to have any life-sustaining efforts when she is dying. While in your ED, she develops an arrhythmia and her heart stops beating. One health care provider starts cardiopulmonary resuscitation (CPR) and wants you to intubate the patient. What would you do and why?

_____

_____

_____

_____

_____

Advance directives and living wills are legal documents patients can use to communicate how they want to be treated if/when they become incapacitated and are dying. These documents are intended to inform providers of the patient's wishes; however, sometimes family members do not agree with the patient's stated directives and want providers to instead do everything possible to keep the patient alive. Conversely, some providers believe that they have an obligation (especially under the biomedical approach) to do everything possible to keep patients alive regardless of the patient's wishes. Such a utilitarian approach presumes that providers know what is best for the patient, even if it is in direct opposition to the patient's stated wishes. Either of these scenarios creates enormous ethical issues for providers. All too often, in 21st-century U.S. health care, patients at the end of their lives are frequently being seen/ treated by providers whom they do not know—usually in EDs, or by hospital-based providers in intensive care units, and so forth; consequently, there is little or no interpersonal relationship between provider and patient during this very important health care decision. Providers need to ask themselves what are patients' expectations regarding their rights and the ethical fulfillment of their wishes for end-of-life care. These answers, combined with an understanding of the theories of rights and justice, should help guide providers' decision making when confronted with an advance directive/living will that may seek a treatment plan (or no treatment) that is different from what the provider would recommend. Clearly, when patients are unable to communicate with providers because of a terminal illness/injury, the provider must decide whether the patient's written directives will be followed, or whether the provider's sense of autonomy and control will supersede the patient's documented decisions.

Reflection 6.7. If you watched *Wit* (2001), as suggested in Chapter 5, then please discuss your thoughts on the "code" scene at the end of the movie when the doctor and nurse clearly have ethical differences of opinion on how the patient's advance directive should be followed. What are the ethical and medical issues to be assessed from a communication perspective?

_____

_____

_____

_____

_____

Reflections (among the possible responses)

6.1. After all your education, clinical training, and health care experience, who do you think is most capable of making decisions about a patient's care, you or the patient? Why?

Although it might seem that a provider is the most capable person to make patient treatment decisions based on the differences in knowledge and experience, this does not account for the fact that we are talking about a patient, not the provider, who is going to endure the consequences of the health care decision. Suppose, for example, you went to jeweler to get your watch repaired and the jeweler decided to fix your watch at a cost of $500 because she or he felt you would not understand the problem or how to fix it—so the jeweler just did what she or he thought was best and you were expected to live with it. Clearly, most Americans would not be happy with such a scenario, we want to know what needs to be done, what it will cost, what the alternatives are, and so forth. However, in health care, the jeweler's example of autonomous decision making was the norm for centuries, and sometimes still is the rule, yet we are talking about a person's health, wellness, and/or survival–not a watch repair. Clearly, health care providers have an obligation to share their knowledge and expertise with their patients, but it is to be hoped that a collaborative decision-making process will ensure that patients feel empowered to participate and are in control of what happens to their body.

6.2. You have a young female patient with a large abdominal mass and the patient wants to know whether the tumor/surgery will keep her from getting pregnant. The scans and tests suggest that the tumor will likely require the removal of at least one ovary and tube, but could require a total hysterectomy and it could be a cancerous tumor, but you will not know until you operate. How will you answer her preoperation question and why?

There are several potential ethical issues to be considered here. One of the most obvious is the theory of rights, which suggests that a patient has a right to truthful and complete information in order to make an informed decision and consent to treatment. However, there is also the provider's concern about frightening, or eliminating the patient's hopes with the details of her condition and possible surgical outcomes. Therefore, a provider might consider trying to circumnavigate around the specific realities of the patient's likely postoperative situation. But the provider's intrapersonal question needs to be: Is this just and right for the patient and will she be able to make a truly informed decision if she does not have the accurate data needed for such a determination? Therefore, the provider might want to present the facts as they are known along with the potential unknowns and how they will impact the patient's fertility. For example, one possible response is "I cannot tell you for certain until after we do the surgery if the tumor and its removal will make you unable to get pregnant or not. And, as we discussed, we will not know until after surgery whether this tumor is a cancer or not. But I can tell you that either way one of your two ovaries will need to be removed. However, if the tumor is also in your uterus or the other tube and/or ovary, then they will have to be removed as well and you would not be able to get pregnant. Based on the test results we have now, I cannot say for certain what will need to be removed; however, I can tell you that we will do our best to not remove your opposite tube, ovary, or uterus. But it is very important that we get all the tumor out and that is our primary goal. Do you have any more questions?" In addition, the provider might also want to use feedback to help determine what the patient heard and assimilated by asking, "I want to be sure I was clear, so can you just tell me what you understand about your tumor, the surgery, and your chances for a postsurgery pregnancy?" This provider–patient interaction uses simple and clear language to describe for the patient the problem, potential risks (cancer and infertility), as well as recognizing the surgical team's goal to both remove the entire tumor but also to preserve the patient's fertility if at all possible. Concomitantly, the provider is using feedback requests to seek further questions, but also to be certain the patient not only heard what the provider said, but was able to assimilate it and communicate it correctly.

6.3. You are working in an emergency department (ED) and a woman who says she is the mother of a 20-year-old patient being treated for alcohol intoxication calls to inquire whether her daughter is in your facility. What do you tell her or do, and why?

Under HIPAA, unless the adult-aged daughter has given permission for her mother to be informed of her treatment (and/or presence in the ED), then you cannot tell the caller anything about the patient or whether she is or is not in your facility. Furthermore, because you have no way to determine whether this is the patient's mother, should the patient give you permission to tell the caller about the patient, you would need the caller to answer some very specific patient-related personal and/or demographic data prior to giving out any information. For example, if the patient has agreed to release information to her mom, then you might ask the woman on the phone for the patient's Social

Security number or another unique identifying piece of information your patient provides that she says only her mother would know (e.g., city where she was born). Again, the goal here is to avoid a situation in which a reporter or friend is pretending to be the patient's mother and whatever information is provided is communicated via social or mass media without the patient's consent.

6.4. Have you been asked to sign a consent form for a procedure/test/service? If so, did you feel fully informed? If not, why not? And if not, did you feel comfortable asking the provider for more information or clarification?

If you have consented to a procedure or service (skin biopsy, MRI, etc.) or even completed the HIPAA form, did the provider explain the document to you? Or were you basically given a form to sign with little or no discussion/explanation? In either case, did the provider take time to explain the procedure and/or service—why it was needed, how it would be done, what the potential benefits and/or risks were, and so forth? If not, how could you be effectively informed to make a decision as to whether you want to proceed, let alone consent to the procedure/service? Although the requirement to have patients sign a consent form may be largely a legal one, the ethical aspects of fully informing the patient with complete and truthful information are just as important to the patient's ability to make decisions and consent to treatment/care.

6.5. How would you respond if you went to a store and nothing you needed had a price on it? So every time you went to buy something, you could not determine whether you could afford it until you were ready to check out? What are the parallels to patient's experiences with tests/procedures/treatment costs and the lack of pricing/billing information prior to a patient's decision making?

Clearly, the customer service and communication problems inherent in such a store policy are obvious. However, when these same issues of informed decision making occur in a health care context, they are not just inconveniences, but ethical quandaries. Patients are being asked to make decisions about their health care without knowing an important determinant—cost. Consequently, we can all agree that without cost issues, our health care decisions might be quite different. We would want the most experienced and successful providers, the most effective diagnostic tests, consultations, treatments, and so forth. But for the overwhelming majority of Americans, cost is a limiting factor in their health care decision making. Similarly, the question is also appropriate as to what the provider's role in addressing the cost issue is when sharing information about a patient's illness/injury and/or treatment? Is it sufficient and ethical for a provider to prescribe a drug, for example, without determining with the patient whether it is affordable based on the patient's economic situation? These are the questions that providers need to address in their personal ethical assessments, as well as their provider–patient interactions. How ethical is it for a provider to diagnose and analyze a patient's condition, educate the patient, prescribe treatment, but not discuss the economic impact of the proposed plan with the patient? This is an often underaddressed ethical component of provider–patient communication and yet as health care costs rise, especially patient-related expenditures (e.g., copays, deductibles, and out-of-pocket), it is an increasingly problematic area for patients.

6.6. You are an ED provider treating a patient who has stage IV cancer and has not responded to surgery, chemotherapy, or radiation. The patient has a living will and advance directive that clearly state her desire not to have any life-sustaining efforts when she is dying. While in your ED, she develops an arrhythmia and her heart stops beating. One health care provider starts cardiopulmonary resuscitation (CPR) and wants you to intubate the patient. What would you do and why?

Unfortunately, this is not an uncommon occurrence in modern health care. For many biomedically trained providers, regardless of the underlying illnesses/injuries—their goal is to keep patients alive. As a consequence, they tend to take a more autonomous and utilitarian view of health care delivery and ignore patients' wishes, even those with advance directives and living wills, in order to keep a patient alive. However, if you do not share this utilitarian, autonomous belief and are in the situation mentioned earlier, you will need to decide whether you want to remind the provider of the patient's directive/decisions, or whether you are going to follow the provider's approach and ignore the patient. These are clearly difficult decisions for providers, especially if they are from different professions/disciplines, with distinct roles and/or hierarchies. However, these dialectical tensions (what the patient wants and what the provider in charge wants) are what makes this an ethical dilemma and what requires providers to have intrapersonally assessed, in advance, how they might communicate in such a scenario so that theirs is not an impulse response, but a well-thought-out reaction.

6.7. If you watched Wit *(2001), as suggested in Chapter 5, then please discuss your thoughts on the "code" scene at the end of the movie when the doctor and nurse clearly have ethical differences of opinion on how the patient's advance directive should be followed. What are the ethical and medical issues to be assessed here from a communication perspective?*

In the "code" scene from the movie, the professor has documented her do-not-resuscitate (DNR) wishes to the appropriate providers. And yet, when the physician/researcher finds her in a state of asystole (no heart function), he disregards the patient's wishes, even the nurse's futile efforts to remind him of the patient's rights and decision. Clearly, this physician chose to act autonomously and ignore the patient's directives, rights, and any sense of justice. His communication behaviors were clearly provider-centric, paternalistic, masculine gendered, and authoritarian. In contrast, the nurse was patient focused, aware of the patient's rights and how unjust the resuscitation efforts were. These provider–provider interactions demonstrate that ethical dilemmas can be perceived differently based on a person's values, beliefs, and goals.

The physician–provider in this movie was clearly focused on keeping his patient alive for further research value at any cost. The nurse–provider, in contrast, was concerned with helping the patient have the best quality of death possible under the circumstances. Consequently, the two providers communicated based on their diverse perspectives. In the end, the patient's wishes were ignored and the physician–provider's unilateral decisions were followed. It is important to remind yourselves as providers that decisions—ethical, clinical, philosophical, and so forth—are all impacted by our intra- and interpersonal communication as well as our values and beliefs.

Skills Exercise

Try out your ability to discuss difficult topics and ethical decision making with older friends of family members. Read the "advance directives" information at the U.S. National Library of Medicine (see Bibliography). Armed with this understanding of advance directives and living wills, have a conversation with two or more older adults about their knowledge of these documents. Ask them what they know about each and also whether they have completed one or both for their end-of-life decisions. If anyone you speak with is unclear or unaware of these health communication/end-of-life care options, please take time to educate the person about his or her rights to make these decisions while they are healthy enough to do so. In addition, if needed, also inform the person about advance directives and living wills and the differences in the two and how your friend/family member can create his or her own and who should be given a copy.

Video Discussion Exercise

Analyze the video

- *Miss Evers' Boys* (1997)

Interactive Simulation Exercise

Pagano, M. (2015). *Communication case studies for health care professionals: An applied approach* (2nd ed.). New York, NY: Springer Publishing Company.

- Chapter 5, "Autonomy Is a Myth" (pp. 45–54)
- Chapter 29, "You Posted What on Facebook?" (pp. 283–290)
- Chapter 32, "You'll Feel Better Recovering at Home" (pp. 309–318)

Health Care Issues in the Media

Escalating price of pharmaceutical products
https://www.youtube.com/watch?v=L-U1MMa0SHw

Informed consent and patients' cells
http://www.nytimes.com/2015/12/30/opinion/your-cells-their-research-your-permission.html

Health Communication Outcomes

There are many intersections of health care delivery and ethical decision making/behaviors. However, this chapter has addressed several common ethical-communication-related scenarios: provider autonomy, truth telling, confidentiality, informed consent, health care economics, and quality of life/ death. Providers need to remember that although their education and expertise clearly offers them unique insights into patient's health care/wellness issues—providers are not the sole arbiters of health care decision making. In an emergency, it is often critical for providers to make autonomous decisions. However, for the overwhelming majority of provider–patient communication and decision making the patient has rights that need to be recognized and ethically honored. In addition, justice would also dictate that providers have an ethical obligation to be truthful and complete in their information sharing and prognostic assessments. It is impossible to expect patients to make empowered, collaborative decisions if they are not given complete and unbiased information with which to make their judgments. Similarly, from the perspectives of legal rights and justice, patients need to be able to trust that providers will ethically honor patients' confidentiality. Although HIPAA laws require it, providers' ethics should assure that no patient information is shared with anyone without the patient's permission. Furthermore, patients have legal and ethical rights and expectations related to informed consent for tests, procedures, and services. Therefore, providers must assure that they not just obtain a patient's signed consent, but that the patient was carefully, thoroughly, and truthfully informed about the planned surgery and so forth using language that the patient could both understand and assimilate. And that the patient's questions and concerns were carefully addressed and effectively answered. And although providers only have some bearing on the economics of patient's care (their fees for example), nonetheless, the provider is the person ordering the tests, procedures, hospitalizations, and so forth. Therefore, we can ask whether the provider bears some responsibility for helping the patient identify the costs associated with the planned treatment, tests, and diagnosis—in order to determine whether he or she can afford them? Finally, providers have ethical obligations to not just consider "curative" approaches, especially for terminally ill individuals, but quality-of-life issues as well. From both theory of rights and theory of justice perspectives, provider–patient communication needs to include discussions of the impact treatment plans will have on patients' quality of life and/or death. As opposed to a biomedical approach that encourages any and all treatments regardless of the likelihood for success, a more ethical undertaking would be to truthfully and completely share information with patients that details the advantages and disadvantages—from both clinical and quality-of-life foci—of various decisions. The role of ethical communication in clinical practice is critical to informed and collaborative decision making, but also to enhancing provider–patient interpersonal relationships and trust.

■ REFERENCE

Skloot, R. (2010). *The immortal life of Henrietta Lacks*. New York, NY: Crown.

■ BIBLIOGRAPHY

Ahronheim, J., Moreno, J., & Zuckerman, C. (2000). Ethics in clinical practice. In *A theory of clinical ethics* (2nd ed., pp. 17–51). Gaithersburg, MD: Aspen.

Brown, J. (2004). Involuntary psychiatric commitment. In G. Pence (Ed.), *Classic cases in medical ethics* (4th ed., pp. 369–394). Boston, MA: McGraw-Hill.

Degrazia, D., Mappes, T., & Ballard J. (2010). *Biomedical ethics* (7th ed.). Boston, MA: McGraw-Hill.

Edelin, K. (2004). Abortion. In G. Pence (Ed.), *Classic cases in medical ethics* (4th ed., pp. 123–151). Boston, MA: McGraw-Hill.

Lo, B. (2013). *Resolving ethical dilemmas: A guide for clinicians* (5th ed.). Philadelphia, PA: Lippincott, Williams & Wilkins.

U.S. National Library of Medicine. (2015). *Advance directives*. Retrieved from https://www.nlm.nih.gov/medlineplus/advancedirectives.html#cat51

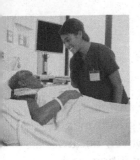

CHAPTER 7

Capitalism, Health Care, and Health Communication

For the purpose of this text, we are going to use the following as working definitions:

- *Acute care:* The philosophical/American approach to health care delivery, whereby most patients are seen for acute/current health care problems, including chronic conditions—not prevention; focuses on finding the immediate issues causing the patient's condition and fixing it

- *Capitalism:* American economic driver in which the primary goal of for-profit organizations is to make a profit and the goal of nonprofit and not-for-profit institutions is to strive to generate as much income as possible

- *Dialectical tension:* Two opposing forces that may be present in various roles, responsibilities, and/or relationships

- *Electronic medical/health records (EMR/EHR):* An electronic format (channel) used to document both patients' health care (past, family, and current) and as an effort to control health care spending

- *Managed care:* A health care procedure/policy instituted by most health insurance companies and Medicare that seeks to reduce costs and improve health care delivery, vis-à-vis third-party oversight of medical decision making and approval for tests, treatments, hospitalizations, and so forth

- *Preventive care:* Cultural and philosophical attitudes that put a premium on health care that is focused on long-term prophylaxis for children and adults; seeks to increase provider–patient collaboration, communication, and information exchanges

■ CAPITALISM, TECHNOLOGY, AND SPECIALIZATION

In the 21st century, health care in America is more of a capitalistic enterprise than ever before. It is the second largest expenditure in the U.S. government's annual budget and provides more than 10 million jobs. However, because so much of health care is viewed from a business model, competition, technology, specialization, and incomes are major drivers. As will be discussed in this and other chapters, the constant evolution of technology in U.S. health care—from the first x-ray machine, microscope, and surgical suite, to today's magnetic resonance imaging devices, robotic surgical apparatuses, and pharmacogenomics—the costs of developing these approaches have increased astronomically. As technology evolved, so too did the belief that specialists would be needed to properly order, use, and interpret these new technological advances. Consequently, another cost driver has been the addition of a wide variety of provider specialists: surgeons, radiologists, ophthalmologists, oncologists, and so forth. However, with a more specialized, technological, and business model approach to health care, not only have economics been impacted, but interpersonal and health communication have as well.

One of the important communication aspects of being a "specialist" is that by definition someone who is "special" is different than others. Therefore, even among other providers, specialists are often perceived as unique based on their education and board certification as a specialist (MD/DO [doctor

> **Reflection 7.1.** How would you perceive the impact of the increases in technology and specialization on health communication and why?
>
> _____
>
> _____
>
> _____
>
> _____
>
> _____

of osteopathy], physician assistant [PA], advanced practice registered nurse [APRN], RN). So a gastroenterologist MD is primarily viewed as an expert in gastrointestinal disorders and sees only patients with related illnesses and is compensated based on his or her specialty. However, health care professionals and insurers are not the only cultures/cocultures that perceive specialists differently than if they were general or family practitioners. Patients also typically view specialists as holding different strata in the health care field. Therefore, if patients who already feel undereducated compared to most health care providers, do not share the specialists' language/terminology, and see distinctions between providers who are specialists and those who are not, these patients are less likely to take an active role in their care/decision making; question the specialist's rationale, diagnosis, and/or treatment recommendations; and/or engage in interpersonal communication/relationship building with someone who is perceived as dissimilar from themselves.

Specialists, therefore, need to be cognizant of these perceptions if they want to encourage dialogues, both with other providers (from different disciplines) and also with patients. Although the realities of a specialist's education, experience, expertise, and certification may be obvious, a specialist who wants to encourage information exchanges, interpersonal communication, and relationship building will need to exercise great care in his or her verbal and nonverbal behaviors. The more a specialist uses language and nonverbal cues to appear more similar to all members of the health care culture, as well as the larger culture, the more likely it is that the interactants will feel similar to him or her and want to collaborate and/or share in the decision making and information exchanges. However, this desire to appear more similar for enhanced provider–provider and provider–patient communication is dialectically opposed to what specialists attempt to do for provider–insurer communication. In order to maximize their reimbursement for consultations, procedures, treatments, and so forth, specialists need to demonstrate verbally and nonverbally to insurers that they are credible experts in their fields. This role of insurers in determining not just which providers will be compensated for their services, but also the differences in compensation based on specialization, helps to contribute to the escalating costs in today's health care and to future providers choosing to specialize versus going into family/general practice areas. Thus, the role of insurers in health care not only markedly influences providers' compensation and career choice, but also the delivery of patient care and the diminishing amount of provider/specialist autonomy.

■ MANAGING HEALTH CARE

Prior to the 1980s in America, health care providers—predominantly physicians—practiced autonomously. They made decisions about patients' health care, diagnosis, and treatments—with whatever patient input was provided/encouraged/allowed, but almost entirely without input from insurers. Consequently, if, during the first three quarters of the 20th century, a provider felt a patient needed a diagnostic test/hospitalization, an elective procedure (cholecystectomy/gall bladder removal), or treatment plan (e.g., physical therapy, medications)—the provider would order whatever he or she felt was needed and bill the patient's insurer (private or Medicare) after the fact. Although these behaviors offered providers the autonomy to make decisions quickly and almost entirely independently—they also resulted in exponentially increasing U.S. health care costs (nationally, organizationally, and individually). Therefore, in the 1980s, American insurers and the federal government started a new, more business-like approach to reducing health costs—managed care.

There are microlevels of managed care, in which organizations insure members who only access the organization's highly regulated/managed system, to macrolevels in which any insured member agrees that his or her provider, except in an emergency, will get approval/permission for any care prior to billing for it. Therefore, managed care in 21st-century America has markedly reduced provider's decision-making autonomy. For example, 20 to 25 years ago, if a patient with insurance came to his or her provider with an acute episode of nontraumatic, low-back pain, he or she might have been sent for a CT scan, or even a surgical consult. However, in 2016, if such a patient is seen, the provider would need to get approval for either the scan or the consult and justify to the case manager at the patient's insurance company why either of these are the most effective plan of care. Typically, however, the case manager will likely recommend that the prescribing provider try physical therapy and reduced lifting for several weeks before a reassessment. The differences in these two approaches to patient care are often not based on the individual patient's condition or provider, but on the insurance company's statistical database that shows the most cost-effective approaches for similar type patient complaints.

Reflection 7.2. What if you are a patient and your provider recommends a treatment plan and your insurance company says that you need to do something different (or pay for the initial plan yourself)? How do you feel about the health care you are receiving (from the provider and insurer)? How does this reality potentially impact your perception of the provider, as well as the value of a provider–patient relationship and interpersonal communication?

_____

_____

_____

_____

_____

Consequently, managed care resulted from an effort to control health care costs (for employers, employees, insurers, and the federal and state governments) vis-à-vis the micromanagement of treatments and services patients can receive. As noted previously, for the wealthiest Americans in the top tier of U.S. health care access, this is not an issue, but for the overwhelming majority of citizens in this country—regardless of having private or government-sponsored health insurance—a person at an insurance company is likely managing their treatment decisions. As you can surmise, this creates a series of communication obstacles for both providers and patients. First, providers are often required to (or have a staff member) communicate with a wide variety of case managers at private and/or government insurers depending on the patient and his or her health insurance, problem, needs, or diagnosis. Second, many patients do not realize they have agreed to allow their health insurance company full access to their medical/health information (without that agreement they cannot get health insurance reimbursement). Finally, for a majority of patients, there is still confusion about who is making the final decision about their health care—the patient, provider, or insurer. All too often, because it is insurers who control the payments for services, they have the ultimate decision making regarding the patient's care. Consequently, managed care can lead to health communication frustration, uncertainty, and hostility. Providers must spend time for which they are not compensated, trying to persuade insurers to approve the provider's treatment plan. Patients are unsure whether the insurer's use of managed care is patient focused or economics based and therefore not in the patient's best interest. In addition, the ability of case managers, often not true peers of the patient's provider (not an MD/DO, PA, APRN, etc.), usually not board certified in the provider's specialty, and sometimes not even health care professionals, to not only assess the patient's condition without ever examining him or her, but to overrule the provider's decisions seems unreasonable. Therefore, managed care can be seen as minimizing, or eliminating, both the provider's and the patient's sense of autonomy in health care decision making. However, managed care is not the only outside influence that potentially creates an ineffective communication exchange between providers and patients.

Reflection 7.3. Read the article by Pagano (2010) in the References section at the end of this chapter and discuss how you think conflict of interest and bias might impact provider–patient communication and patient treatment outcomes.

_____

_____

_____

_____

_____

■ CAPITALISM AND MEDICINE—INFLUENCE AND BIAS

As discussed earlier, health care is an economic driver in the U.S. economy and as such has made many corporations very wealthy. It is also important to note that even though many American hospitals (or health systems) are non-profit organizations, that does not mean that executives in those facilities cannot be very well paid. For example, numerous chief executive officers (CEOs) of nonprofit hospitals/health systems have annual million, or multi-million, dollar salaries, and with benefits and perks can earn over $2 or $3 million a year. It is important for health providers, regardless of their professions, to understand the impact of capitalism on modern U.S. health care delivery. It should not be surprising that the cost of health care in America, coupled with enormous profits for private health care organizations, CEOs, and others in nonprofit hospitals/health systems, could impact the interpersonal and organizational communication between providers and their institutions as well as their attitudes and perceptions of the organization.

Perhaps some of the most destructive—from communication and ethical perspectives—aspects of the capitalistic impact on health communication, trust, and information sharing are conflict of interest and bias. For example, it is not uncommon to hear both providers and/or patients jokingly remark,

Communicator A: "Why did the provider order that?"

Communicator B: "Beats me, must be time for a boat payment."

This exchange emphasizes some of the conflict-of-interest issues that plague providers, organizations, and patients. On one hand, the sarcastic remark implies that a provider would order a test, procedure, or treatment for reasons other than the patient's illness/injury/wellness—to make money off of his or her professional recommendation. However, this brief commentary also reminds us about the role socioeconomic status plays in provider–patient and provider–provider communication and interpersonal relationships. Specifically, the provider in this example is not just making money—unethically, vis-à-vis a conflict of interest, but is also wealthy enough to afford a boat. Although it seems likely that the overwhelming majority of health care providers in America are not prescribing treatments, tests, or other services in order to make money off of them—it is true that with managed care restrictions and micromanagement of providers' decisions, U.S. health care providers' incomes have decreased—especially among nonspecialists (Jauhar, 2015). It is important for providers to be vigilant about their patient communication and use their interpersonal relationships to help educate and explain the reasons for all tests, procedures, and services.

One of the areas in health care that has generated numerous concerns about conflict of interest is the role of providers in pharmaceutical drug development, marketing, education, and publication. Because providers are often paid employees/consultants for the pharmaceutical companies whose products the providers are researching/presenting, there are fears that the monetary aspects of the provider–manufacturer relationship could lead to misinformation, obfuscation, or biased recommendations. However, capitalism, conflict of interest, and bias are not just related to provider–patient and provider–provider interactions.

As has been reported by the Food and Drug Administration (FDA), numerous pharmaceutical and medical device manufacturers have misrepresented, miscommunicated, or deceived the FDA, providers, and patients with their research, marketing, and advertisements (Pagano, 2010). Again, based on the potential economic benefits of a new drug or device, it is possible for a provider or patient to receive misinformation related to bias or conflict of interest by either the organization and/or its employees and consultants. Therefore, it behooves both providers and patients to carefully assess all health-related information and not assume that it is correct just because it has been peer reviewed and/or approved. The impact of financial gain in health care delivery creates major communication issues for providers and patients related to health care education, risk assessment, and accurately informed decision making. The economic realities of 21st-century health care and their associated impact on provider–patient, provider–provider, and provider–organization communication are evident in all aspects of the delivery system.

■ FROM A CLINICAL TO A BUSINESS MODEL

Although there are clear differences between the biomedical and biopsychosocial models of health care delivery, they are both similar in that their goals are to improve the patient's condition (from an illness/injury focus and/or a wellness/quality-of-life approach). However, at the macrolevel of health care in U.S. culture, we have evolved from a largely scientific, clinical-based approach to a business-centric model where profits and loss, dominate almost all major organizational decisions. Today, pharmaceutical manufacturers are choosing to research more "me too" (newer versions of current prescription) drugs, than risk developing new treatment modalities. Similarly, hospitals are competing with neighboring institutions by duplicating technologies and services that cost millions of dollars, rather than negotiating a way to share devices and minimize the competitive marketing. Furthermore, many hospitals and health systems are purchasing provider practices in order to impact admissions, but also to allow patient billing of insurers at the hospital, not the private office rate. This effort to focus organizational goals more on the business aspect of health care rather than on clinical characteristics is creating unique professional choices for health care providers.

With the increasing costs (money and time) associated with private practice, malpractice insurance/liability, and managed care—it should not be surprising that nearly half of all physicians and most other providers now are employees of hospitals and/or other health systems. This evolution in provider practice also raises conflict-of-interest/bias concerns from a patient's perspective about whether employees are ordering tests and services to meet some institutional quota or bonus opportunity versus what the patient truly needs. In addition, from a provider viewpoint, one of the current ways in which hospitals and other health service organizations assess their impact on their customers/patients is through postvisit surveys. One of the major public relations tools of this type is the Press Ganey satisfaction survey sent to patients after visits to an emergency department (ED) or after a hospital stay. The data from these assessments are then frequently used by hospitals to encourage providers to change behaviors, shorten wait times, and/or alter patients' perceptions of their organizational experiences. Although it can be argued that feedback from customers or patients is important information to use in analyzing how target audiences perceive an organization and/or its employees, to use wait times for an ED as a way to measure a provider's performance is problematic at best and nonsensical at worst.

As we have discussed, EDs in 21st-century health care are the only access point for many Americans. Although it is true that the uninsured often have nowhere else to go for health care—acute or chronic—it is also true that most insured and uninsured patients have no other options for acute care after office hours, on weekends, and over holidays. As private practice has evolved in this culture, providers are not paid for phone consultations with patients; however, their recommendations, treatment plans, prescriptions, and so forth, are all subject to malpractice and as they are not examining the patient when making these decisions—they face increasing liability risks if they choose to consult with patients after hours over the phone. And the costs (time, money, legal risk, and so forth) to see a patient in the office or the patient's home after normal business hours are prohibitive. Therefore, most patients, insured and uninsured, who seek to speak with or see their private provider outside the normal office hours are instructed to go to an ED if they cannot wait for the next available appointment. Therefore, ED wait times are a function, not just of the time spent with an ED provider, but of a health care system that uses the ED as its sanctuary for anyone wanting to be seen for any problem 24/7/365. As a result, ED providers frequently only have one way to shorten wait times— spend less time interacting with ED patients. However, as you might imagine, patients who wait 2 to 3 hours or more to see a provider are generally not happy to begin with and then to get less time than expected to tell their story, gather information, and feel properly evaluated makes these customers not only unhappy about the wait time, but also about the services they received or did not receive. And they use the Press Ganey surveys as their feedback tool for communicating their displeasure with the institution to hospital administrators. These administrators then provide this feedback to their providers and "encourage" them in one way or another to change the problem (which is of course generally not something they can control—who comes to an ED, why they come, or whether they need to be seen in an ED). These efforts by hospitals to improve customers' feedback often create more organization–provider communication problems because providers feel they have no control and yet they are being held responsible for the situation and rewarded or punished based on the survey results. In fact, the use of customer surveys without a thoughtful assessment of the context, culture, communication, and shared goals further highlights use of a business approach versus a clinical/social science understanding of the problems from patient, provider, and organizational perspectives. Furthermore, this business focus in modern health care has impacted other areas of interpersonal communication—the patient's record.

■ THE ECONOMICS OF EMRs AND EHRs

Perhaps nowhere is the negative impact of economics and a business model approach to health care delivery more obvious than in the development and regulated usage of EMRs/EHRs. Although some use the terms *EMR* and *EHR* interchangeably, for the purpose of this text, EMR will be used for provider-created documents and EHR will be considered self-record keeping

Reflection 7.4. What are some of the pros and cons of electronic medical record (EMR) usage in health communication and health care?

_____

_____

_____

_____

_____

(typically on a website) by patients. It is true that there were numerous problems with pen-and-paper medical records, including:

- Legibility
- Brevity
- Inconsistent data (quantity and quality)
- Storage and retrieval issues
- Timeliness

One of the major problems with hand-written medical records was the difficulty presented by providers' handwriting. And without effective written documentation, the record could not meet its major goal of communicating information from one provider to others. One of the efforts in the latter half of the 20th century to overcome legibility and penmanship issues in medical records was the use of dictation and transcription. However, this process and format, which sought to improve the documentation, especially in postoperative, pathology, and radiology reports, was both financially challenging for the institution and still depended on the provider reviewing the typed report and revising it as needed for accuracy. The problem with this process was that providers frequently did not review the report. They would sign it and only later find out there were significant mistakes, misspelled words, and typos (e.g., "left kidney removed," when it should have been "right"). And if providers did not do their dictation in a timely manner, the record would be even more delayed and, until complete, the hospital/office could not submit the appropriate documentation to insurers to get compensated for services provided. But the problems with handwritten records went beyond just legibility issues.

Although there were clearly templates for documenting various procedures: Histories and Physicals, Reports, Progress Notes, and so forth, providers had no real oversight—unless there was a legal issue—to assure that the record provided clear, complete documentation of the who, what, why, where, when, and how for each entry. Even the standard template for a progress note (subjective, objective, assessment, and plan [SOAP]) could end up being as ineffectively communicated as:

S: T. 99.6 (o)

O: erythema at wound margins

A: probable superficial wound infection

P: incision and drain (I & D), recheck tomorrow

Although the author of such a note could argue that the basics of his or her exam are reported here, the reader has to go elsewhere to determine what the patient was being seen for. It is true that the subjective information communicates the likelihood that the patient does not have a significant systemic infection based on the lack of a fever, but there is more information about how the patient feels (subjective) that would have helped. In addition, objectively the wound (undescribed) is reported to show signs of a localized infection (erythema = redness), and the provider plans to I & D it and recheck it the next day. It would not have taken but a few minutes longer to supply additional information for the reader (the major reason for writing a medical record) that would have eliminated the need to seek out more details earlier in the record, or consult a different provider, or the author, by phone or face to face (F2F), to learn more about the patient's condition. Examples like this were used to highlight the need for more consistent, informative, and structured medical records that were not just legible, but served their intended purpose and goal—informing readers about the patient's illness/injury/examination/findings, and so forth.

Reportedly, in an effort to improve medical record documentation and communication, the federal government created requirements for the development and implementation of EMRs in U.S. hospitals; to ensure compliance the government tied Medicare reimbursement to hospitals' adoption of EMRs. However, although the potential for improved health communication exchange was clearly possible with effective EMR development and usage, the organizational change (across U.S. health care institutions) was independent, lacked important input and feedback from health care providers as well as writing and reading scholars, and appeared to be more economic focused than clinical/patient centered.

First and foremost, without leadership, hospitals and other health care organizations set out independently to work with EMR software developers to create proprietary EMR systems that could be used within a health care system, but not outside of it. Therefore, the portability benefits of having one EMR for a patient, which could be accessed at any U.S. health care institution, were not possible with the every-institution-for-itself model of EMR development. Similarly, with the competitive, capitalistic business approach to U.S. health care, there was little to no sharing of information or experiences between hospitals and health systems. So the problems faced by one institution might be also seen at a competitor across town, but because of the business approach the two organizations did not communicate with each other and both suffered the consequences and costs. In addition, the expense of creating massive EMR software programs on an ad hoc basis meant that each institution/health system generally had to discover its own needs and how to attain them. Some hospitals spent millions of dollars on their EMR development, whereas health systems spent hundreds of millions, and still are able to share only with the three or four hospitals and private provider offices in their system and no one else—except insurers. The ability to share data with insurers was the one underlying consistent requirement of all EMRs. They cannot share clinical information across health care institutions/providers, but they *all* can share billing and patient information with insurers.

Once again, the capitalistic, business aspect of 21st-century heath care delivery demonstrates that the common denominator in EMR communication is organization–insurer, not provider–provider, provider–organization, or provider–patient. Furthermore, with a major focus on documentation for billing and reimbursement, very little research/analysis seems to be have been done regarding how to minimize the negative impact on provider–patient interactions with EMR usage. Consequently, providers today often access the EMR in an exam room, paying more attention to the keyboard and monitor than to the patient. Similarly, providers frequently position the desktop, laptop, tablet, or computer on wheels (COW), in between them and the patient, or worse, in a position where the provider's back is facing the patient while the provider types in the EMR. In hospitals, patients and families often complain that the nursing staff spends more time on the computer than with the patient. The requirements for documentation, especially to assure that billing/reimbursement requirements have been fulfilled, assure that more information is provided than in written records, but at the same time many hospital providers complain that too many EMR authors merely copy and paste a lengthy entry from 1 day to the next. So that it appears from the record that a patient with pneumonia had a rectal exam 6 days in a row—with no explanation for why one was necessary on a daily basis. The potential benefits of an EMR that can be both clearly and concisely authored with accurate information that helps all users understand the who, what, where, why, when, and how of a patient's condition, progress, procedure, and so forth will remain elusive until there is a concerted effort to create EMRs that are both patient centered and economically appropriate. But in addition, EMRs need to be part of a national, secure database system that can be accessed, with the patient's permission, by providers across the country. However, EMRs were legislated and regulated based on the reality that we have an illness-focused, rather than a wellness-centered health care system.

■ REWARDS FOR TREATING, NOT FOR PREVENTING, ILLNESS/INJURY

Based on the current culture of health care—predominantly biomedical, technology driven, and operating under a capitalistic business model—the rewards for health-related organizations and providers are based on treating illnesses/injuries, not preventing them. For example, if you are a manufacturer of a pharmaceutical or medical device company, do you think there is more money in curing a disease, preventing it, or treating it? As you likely have deduced, selling 30 pills a month for 30 years is much more profitable than developing a way to prevent hypertension. Similarly, it is much more profitable to sell a knee replacement that may work effectively for 10 years or less, than it is to find a way to protect knees from arthritis and injuries. And hospitals are paid for treating ill and injured patients and not for keeping them well. But in the current health care culture, providers are also rewarded by being paid for every patient visit, procedure, test, and so on, not for keeping patients well and only requiring occasional prevention evaluations.

Historically, the culture of health care has evolved from a time when there was little or nothing understood about the etiology of disease processes or of various health risks—therefore, acute and chronic care were the only real possibilities in ancient Egypt and Greece and in the medieval and pre–industrial revolution world. However, as knowledge and science evolved, instead of focusing on the patient and preventing illnesses and injuries, the trillions of dollars spent annually on 21st-century American health care are predominantly required to cover the costs of treating diseases and trauma (that result from a lack of prevention focus, education, and an economic incentive).

Reflection 7.5. As a health care provider who is paid by insurers, patients, and/or a health care organization based on the number of patients you see, the tests you order and interpret, and the procedures you perform—how do you think the current disease-focused incentivizing process will impact your provider–patient communication and potentially your decision making/recommendations? (see Jauhar, 2015)

_____

_____

_____

_____

_____

Based on the economic realities of the current disease/injury-focused health care system, patient communication clearly is at risk. If providers (as well as health care organizations) are compensated for treatments—not prevention—then it only makes sense that health care services are going to be focused on maximizing the ways to be paid—while still trying to effectively treat the patient. For example, if you need a routine colonoscopy, you likely will have to see the provider for an office visit and then at a later date have your colonoscopy. One of the reasons, if not the major reason, is that providers cannot get paid for the "office visit" if it is on the same day as the procedure. It has been argued that gastroenterologists and other providers need to discuss and educate the patient about the procedure in advance—thereby justifying the need for the office visit. However, if the patient was the focus of health care, then why couldn't a method be devised that addressed the clinical, economic, and legal concerns and provided an opportunity for provider–patient communication with less impact on the patient (e.g., phone call or e-mail). Then, prior to the procedure and anesthesia, the provider and patient could briefly discuss any questions, clarifications, and so forth. In this communication model, the patient's time and needs are the focus—rather than the provider's, insurer's, and so on. The problems for providers who wish to use such a model today are:

1. They will not be paid for either the phone/e-mail information exchange

2. Insurers see duplication of billing when providers charge for separate office/procedure fees that occur during the same visit

3. Malpractice attorneys may question the legal risks of educating patients by e-mail or phone (even though they can be sent the same printed instructions they are given in F2F office visits and patients can still seek clarifications and more information—regardless of how the initial exchange occurs)

As colonoscopy is a preventive measure, it would seem that making it as convenient (time and effort) and cost-effective as possible would be a key goal. However, because the health care system/culture is based on a disease-focused model, prevention is economically "treated" like an illness/injury. Therefore, if you want to take a patient-centered, biopsychosocial approach to prevention, as well as disease/injury diagnosis and treatment, you may frequently find yourself in a dialectical dilemma between billing/payment for service and quality-of-life care. Clearly, as providers need to earn a living, pay bills, and so forth, the issue for 21st-century health care professionals is, are you willing to try and change the health care culture by, whenever possible, making your patients, prevention, and their quality of life the focus of your provider–patient interpersonal communication, goals, values, and behaviors?

Reflections (among the possible responses)

7.1. How would you perceive the impact of increases in technology and specialization on health communication and why?

There are many ways in which the evolution in technology and provider/health care specialization have impacted provider–patient, provider–provider, and provider–organization health communication. As technology exponentially increased in health care delivery over the past century, there was both a commensurate escalation in health care costs for equipment and services, but also a surge in the education and expansion of provider specialists to manage the equipment, assess patients related to the discipline, and interpret the results. As costs, technology, and specializations increased, providers chose specialties over primary care, which not only impacted provider–patient communication, but also affected access to care; fewer primary care providers led to inappropriate use of EDs, specialists, and less continuity of care—all of which negatively impact effective health communication exchanges.

7.2. What if you are a patient and your provider recommends a treatment plan and your insurance company says that you need to do something different (or pay for the initial plan yourself)? How do you feel about the health care you are receiving (from the provider and insurer)? How does this reality potentially impact your perception of the provider, as well as the value of a provider–patient relationship and interpersonal communication?

As a patient who is told by your provider that you need one type of treatment and your insurance company/case manager wants a different approach, you are likely to feel confused, distrustful, and/or insignificant. Because most patients believe that their providers are making the best recommendations for their health, it is often very worrisome when his or her recommendations are overridden by a case manager you do not know, have never seen, and who has not examined/communicated with you. Similarly, the fact that your provider's recommendation was not just called into question, but rejected, likely will make you curious about the provider's assessment, decision making, and recommendations. Consequently, providers should recognize a potential conflict (dialectical tension) between the patient's diagnosis/treatment needs and insurance plan's case management algorithms and discuss in advance with the patient the possibility of a different approach if required. In so doing, the provider can both prepare the patient for a change in plans and also explain to the patient that although either option will likely work, there was a reason why the provider chose the plan that was recommended. This interpersonal communication should help reassure the patient and further the provider–patient relationship. In addition, if the provider's plan is altered, the patient is more likely to question the case manager's reasons for altering the recommendation (without seeing/talking with the patient) rather than the provider.

7.3. Read the article by Pagano (2010) listed in the References section at the end of this chapter and discuss how you think conflict of interest and bias might impact provider–patient communication and patient treatment outcomes.

Some of the ways that conflict of interest and bias might impact provider–patient communication and treatment outcomes revolve around the role that provider–consultants play in pharmaceutical and medical device research, development, testing, publication, and promotion. Because the manufacturer has a vested financial interest in the product, as well as the paid provider-consultants, it makes the accuracy, completeness, and analysis of the information presented questionable and may call the "spokes-provider's/ thought-leader's" credibility into question. Historically, numerous pharmaceutical products and medical devices have been touted as safe and effective by manufacturers and consultants, even approved by the FDA, only later to find that the information presented in research, marketing, and/ or provider continuing education was duplicitous, inaccurate, or fallacious. Patients and providers can only see this pattern of miscommunication as

problematic in terms of treatment, decision making, product/manufacture/
spokes-provider trust, and an effective provider–patient health communication exchange.

*7.4. What are some of the pros and cons of electronic medical record (EMR) usage
related to health communication and health care?*

As pointed out in this chapter, some of the pros of EMR usage include
(a) legibility; (b) consistency (within a hospital/health care system/organiza-
tion); (c) timeliness of documentation; and (d) ease of access (within a hospital/
health care system/organization). However, there are several problems associated with EMR usage, especially related to provider–patient and provider–
provider health communication: (a) authors are limited in many aspects to a
checklist response, not a narrative; (b) documentation is dependent on accurate
and specific information (not copied and pasted responses entry after entry);
(c) providers' documentation in EMR may interfere verbally and nonverbally
with the provider–patient interaction (add noise to the channel); (d) providers'
need to document in the EMR may negatively impact the provider–patient
interpersonal relationship, especially if EMR is viewed by the patient as more
important to the provider than the patient; (e) EMR is not geographically available across institutions.

*7.5. As a health care provider who is paid by insurers, patients, and/or a health
care organization, based on the number of patients you see, the tests you order
and interpret, and the procedures you perform—how do you think the current
disease-focused incentivizing process will impact your provider–patient communication and potentially your decision making/recommendations (see Jauhar, 2015)?*

One of the dialectical tensions that providers must deal with on a daily basis is
the issue between billing for patient's services and what tests, exams, and procedures are truly needed. For example, you are seeing a 50-year-old patient
for a cough and congestion; based on your exam do you really need a chest
x-ray (CXR) and EKG to check for a pneumonia or cardiac etiology for the
chest congestion—both of which you can bill extra for? Or do you treat the
patient for the upper respiratory illness (URI) you suspect and only bill for
an office visit? Based on the patient's age and symptoms, you likely could
make the case for ruling out a cardiac or pulmonary etiology for the chest
congestion and, therefore, need the two tests, which, if done in your office,
you can bill for separately—and also for *each* of your interpretations of the
CXR and EKG. Consequently, you will need to decide whether you want to
bill the patient's insurance and/or the patient (copay or self-pay) for an office
visit, or an office visit plus a CXR, plus an EKG, plus the assessment of the
CXR and the evaluation of the EKG. As you can see, there is a significant
financial incentive for a provider to do more tests. However, by using the
disease-focused incentive-payment process to drive your decision making

you need to not only question your ethics, but also your relationship with your patient and how you communicate (truth or untruth) about what he or she needs in order to have a reasonable diagnosis and treatment plan. Remember, health communication is more than just the words you use—it includes not only the information you seek and share, but also the veracity of that information sharing and whether or not you are allowing personal financial gain, conflict of interest, and/or bias to inappropriately influence your decision making, patient education, and interpersonal communication/relationships.

Skills Exercise

You are a health care provider who is working in a busy ED or urgent care facility and the wait time to be seen is 2.5 to 3 hours. You are seeing a patient for the first and she is upset about how long the wait was. How would you (verbally and nonverbally) try to communicate to her that in spite of the wait and the packed waiting room, you are going to give her problem/needs your full attention? Consider that your patient takes her car to a repair shop and has to wait for 2.5 hours just to get it looked at. How would you hypothesize such a wait would impact her perception of the organization and the organization's employees? What would you expect the repair organization to do to communicate its understanding of the value of your time (as a customer) and of your unmet expectations for service? What parallels (unmet expectations/frustrations/distrust) do you see for your patient as a customer in the two organizations?

Video Discussion Exercise

Analyze the video

- *John Q* (2002)

Interactive Simulation Exercise

Pagano, M. (2015). *Communication case studies for health care professionals: An applied approach* (2nd ed.). New York, NY: Springer Publishing Company.

- Chapter 15, "Why Do I Have to Wait for an MRI?" (pp. 151–160)
- Chapter 33, "I Only Have 9 Minutes or So" (pp. 319–328)
- Chapter 45, "I Shouldn't Have to Wait; I Have Insurance" (pp. 423–430)

Health Care Issues in the Media

The costs of dying
https://www.youtube.com/watch?v=F6xPBmkrn0g

Health Communication Outcomes

This chapter has explored the impact of capitalism and economic realities on health communication, patients, and the current use of a business model approach to health care delivery. The role of managed care in changing the provider–patient interaction as well as providers' autonomy was described and explained. Furthermore, based on the capitalistic approach to illnesses/injuries in the United States—the potential for conflict of interest and bias by providers and health care organizations is well documented. In addition, the risks of conflict of interest and bias in diagnosis, treatments, products, and services add more uncertainty and mistrust into provider–patient, provider–provider, and provider–organization communication. In order to change the future of health care, providers, patients, and the U.S. culture will need to demand a more patient-centric, quality-of-life, and prevention focus to both health communication and health care delivery.

■ REFERENCES

Jauhar, S. (2015). *Doctored: The disillusionment of an American physician.* New York, NY: Farrar, Straus and Giroux.

Pagano, M. P. (2010). Conflict of interest, bias, and manipulation: Reassessing prescriber education and the Learned Intermediary Doctrine. *Communication Law Review, 10*(2), 30–47. Retrieved from http://commlawreview .org/Archives/CLRv10i2/Conflict%20of%20Interest,%20Bias,%20and%20 Manipulation%20CLR%20v10i2.pdf

■ BIBLIOGRAPHY

Goldsteen, R., & Goldsteen, K. (2013). History of change: From prepaid group medical practice to managed care. In R. Goldsteen & K. Goldsteen (Eds.), *Jonas' introduction to U.S. health care system* (7th ed., pp. 209–232). New York, NY: Springer Publishing Company.

Kassirer, J. (2005). On the take: How medicine's complicity with big business can endanger your health. In J. P. Kassirer (Ed.), *Your doctor's tainted information* (pp. 79–102). Oxford, UK: Oxford University Press.

Shi, L., & Singh, D. (2015). Delivering health care in America: A systems approach. In L. Shi & D. Singh (Eds.), *Managed care and integrated organizations* (6th ed., pp. 335–377). Burlington, MA: Jones & Bartlett.

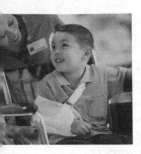

CHAPTER 8

Health Care Organizational Communication

For the purpose of this text, we are going to use the following as working definitions:

- *Human behavior theory:* Theoretical perspective that focuses on the employees and their motivations

- *Interdependent:* Elements of an organization (individual or group) that work independently but contribute collaboratively to assure effective task/goal outcomes

- *Organizational communication:* Information sharing that is internal (employees/members) and external (customers, stakeholders)

- *Scientific management theory:* Theoretical approach to organizing that takes an objective/scientific perspective

- *Stakeholder:* A person or group that contributes to the work and/or goals of an organization, which may be an employee, stockholder, group, or organization; for example, a group of orthopedic surgeons who are not paid by a hospital but who do surgery and treat their patients there, would be nonemployee, group stakeholders

- *Stockholder:* A person or group who owns stock in an organization and expects to earn dividends on his or her or their investment

- *Vender:* A person or group who does business with an organization (e.g., hospital-bed manufacturer)

■ ORGANIZATIONAL COMMUNICATION

At its most basic level, communication is required for organizing. Therefore, the way we think of organizations: family, school, corporation, nonprofit, health care, and so forth, are based on how communication is used to both

143

create the company/entity as well as inform others—internal and external—about its particular mission, values, and goals. Consequently, the way we view one health care organization versus another is based in large part on how it communicates. For example, St. Jude Children's Research Hospital is similar to many other hospitals in its commitment to health care delivery; however, its mission is to research and treat children's illnesses without charging parents for the cost of their child's hospital visits. The Connecticut (CT) Hospice is an inpatient health care organization, but unlike St. Jude, the CT Hospice is organized around the goal of focusing on enhancing dying patients' and their families' quality of life and death. For providers, health care organizations may have similar goals but very distinct values, beliefs, and missions. One hospital might be a nonprofit, whereas another is a for-profit institution. Therefore, providers need to understand the difference between nonprofits—whose goals are to spend whatever income remains after paying bills within the organization (salaries, equipment, construction, etc.) and not have a profit. However, for-profit companies' goals are to make profits (monies remaining after all bills are paid). Generally, both nonprofit and for-profit organizations have stakeholders; however, only for-profit organizations have stockholders who expect to be compensated for their investments.

Reflection 8.1. Think of two organizations (family, school, health care, religious, etc.) of which you are a member. How do you see the communication (internally and externally) being different in the two organizations, from your perspective? How does the internal communication impact your perceptions of the organization? Is one better at communicating internally (with members) than the other? If so, why?

_____

_____

_____

_____

_____

As you have likely surmised, if you are a health care provider who is seeking employment at a health care organization, it would be important to understand whether it is a for-profit or nonprofit institution. The organization's economic focus will tell you a lot about the institution's values, beliefs, and goals—all of which will impact communication—provider–patient, provider–provider, and provider–organization. Keep in mind: All health care organizations are trying to generate income (from services, donations, products, etc.). However, for some businesses/institutions generating maximum income for stockholders and stakeholders is their highest priority. For others, bringing in enough money to cover bills and meet customers/clients/patients' needs is critical. As discussed in Chapter 7, health care in America is predominantly organized using a business approach—making money, regardless of whether it is a for-profit or nonprofit entity. Therefore, whether you intend to work in a hospital, private office, public health clinic, pharmaceutical company, and so on your communication from and with the organization will, in large part, be related to its business/economic goals and values. But the organizational communication realities for providers and patients are related to the theoretical foundations of a health care organization as well as its financial goals.

■ ORGANIZATIONAL COMMUNICATION THEORIES

Throughout history, organizing, maintaining, changing, and succeeding in the development and attainment of group goals fundamentally depended on one constant—communication. Without effective interpersonal, small-group, organizational, and mass communication—organizations cannot succeed. Therefore, as you think about health care organizations (regardless of their mission and/or goals: private, public, for profit, or nonprofit), they are linked by the need for effective communication—internally and externally.

In America, with the industrial revolution and the need to organize individuals to work interdependently, early theorists Frederick Taylor, Henri Fayol, Max Weber, and later Mary Parker Follett and Douglas McGregor, among others proposed a variety of communication approaches. Evolving from a primarily independent, largely agriculture-based, rural society to an urban, codependent coculture required a new approach to organizing and communicating. In health care, for example, prior to 1910, the delivery of health services was frequently at the patient's home/farm or in the provider's office. To move from a largely unorganized health care delivery method to the highly structured system we have today required the communication of the organization's mission, goals, and values, but also its members' roles, responsibilities, status, and hierarchy.

The early organizational theorists proposed that companies should be approached as if they were a machine—with a variety of different parts—all of which work independently but also collaboratively with the rest of the machine to accomplish its goal. The success of the (machine) organization depends on all employees (parts) working interdependently. Just as a car needs wheels, a chassis, seats, steering wheel, engine parts, and so forth all working in a standardized and replaceable way for the car to start, run, stop, and repeat all of those functions—organizations need similar processes and outcomes. Therefore, based on 100-year-old theories, the overwhelming majority of U.S. professional establishments utilize this mechanistic view of organizing in hiring, firing, evolving, brand building, and communicating. As a result, health care providers need to understand the importance of standardization, rules, replaceability, status, and hierarchy in hiring, promotions, and in successfully attaining institutional goals and outcomes.

Reflection 8.2. Why do you think medical, nursing, and physician assistant (PA) schools, for example, have specific, but differing, requirements to be accepted? And why do they not all teach health information from one perspective? How does this illustrate the role of organizational communication in providers' lives from earliest entry into the disciplines/professions?

_____

_____

_____

_____

_____

Have you ever stopped to think about how a hospital is organized? Let's put on our mechanistic lenses and examine how communication impacts the way hospitals are organized and operate.

1. Employees are hired based on their roles.

2. Employees' roles are standardized (administrator, doctor, nurse, tech, custodian, etc.).

3. Employees are replaceable (if one leaves, his or her role is filled by another qualified/standardized person).

4. There are clear policies and procedures—rules—that govern behavior.

5. Hospitals generally follow a vertical hierarchy, communication flows predominantly downward from the board of directors to chief executive officer to medical and nursing directors, and so forth to employees (nurses, doctors, quality control, maintenance, housekeeping, etc.).

6. Status is very apparent in most hospitals: the administration have offices and titles that illustrate this; professions intra- and interprofessionally use titles, licenses, specialization, and so forth to demonstrate their various status distinctions.

While there are countless ways we could deconstruct the organizing of hospitals or other health care institutions, if we just use these six criteria we should readily see how important organizational theories and communication are to the effective operation and goal attainment of health care delivery systems. For example, from a health care organization perspective, it is critical to have standardized roles and responsibilities. Therefore, doctors and nurses clearly do have specific roles and/or are responsibilities for similar, but diverse aspects of health care delivery and patient communication, assessment, and treatment. However, if one RN in the neonatal intensive care unit (NICU) decides she or he wants more money or more vacation time off, the hospital can evaluate that request but not feel coerced to honor those wishes. Because health care providers (MD/DO [doctor of osteopathy], RN, advanced practice registered nurse [APRN], physician assistant [PA], etc.) have standardized education and training that is state/federally regulated and leads to either licensure or certification, most can be replaced based on their profession/certification (cardiologist, orthopedist, NICU RN, etc.). Therefore, as with almost all professional U.S. organizations, standardization and replaceability are critical both to the interdependent nature of 21st-century business/health care goals, but also to the efficacy of human resource management. Consequently, every day new members of a hospital are not just acculturated into the organization, but for the most part seamlessly take over a role and responsibility previously done by someone else. As you can see, and theorists recognized 100 years ago, the benefits of standardization and replaceability for organizations, especially in today's health care system are undeniable. However, over the past 100 years, the more standardized and replaceable health care providers became vis-à-vis consistent, codified, and mandated education and clinical training, the less individualized and autonomous health care providers and institutions have become. If you were a cardiovascular surgeon, operating room nurse, or pump technician in the 1960s and 1970s as this new specialty began to grow—you could communicate your uniqueness and irreplaceability in numerous organizational ways, but definitely in your salary, role, and other demands. However, 50 years later, countless cardiovascular and other specialty physicians, nurses, PAs, and so forth are educated and trained, so while still a prestigious coculture, like most other hospital staff, they are replaceable and therefore now have less power and control related to their unique roles and responsibilities. As you likely have deduced, although the value of standardization and replaceability are crucial for health care organizations, they are less valued by some providers—who still see themselves as independent practitioners who are for the most part irreplaceable. But as we progress with the business model approach to health care in the 21st century, providers are becoming more organizational based than ever before. In fact, the latest trend in modern health care is for hospitals to buy physicians' private practices so that the physicians become hospital employees and the organization can bill the physicians' office patients and/or their insurers at the higher hospital rate for services. But standardization, replaceability, and status are only part of the way communication is used by health care organizations to impact employees' work and goal attainment efforts. Policies, procedures, and rules help impact how a health care organization functions, how providers and others work interdependently, and how information flows throughout the organization.

Research Exercise 8a. Do you know what a hospitalist is and what that role is in modern health care/hospitals? If so, please describe both, if not, please research and describe both. From communication, clinical, and economic perspectives, how do you think the organization uses hospitalists, instead of the patient's provider, to better meet the hospital's goals?

_____

_____

_____

_____

_____

All organizations use rules to help organize employees' behaviors. Those rules in health care organizations are more than just starting and quitting work times, vacation, and so forth, they are most often formal policies and procedures codified in bound (or electronic) volumes that are not just part of the institutional archives, but a required part of new employee orientation, in-service/continuing-education courses and evaluations. In fact, to obtain/maintain national accreditation with The Joint Commission, one of the requirements is well-documented and effectively communicated hospital policies, procedures, and rules. Therefore, one of the more critically important organizational roles/departments for American hospitals is the field of risk management (see Chapter 12). One of the key goals of risk management is to work with the appropriate staff of the hospital to identify potential problems or analyze and strategize solutions for adverse events in order to develop new and/or revised policies and procedures to help avoid future problems/medical errors. Clearly, from a health care organizational perspective, policies, procedures, and codified rules are needed to help members/employees' work interdependently and communicate effectively in order to provide the most safe and productive health care delivery possible. However, as you know, policies, procedures, and rules are only successful in goal attainment, effective patient care, and positive outcomes if employees have read/heard them, assimilated the information, clarified any misperceptions, and follow them. Organizations are constantly reminded that without effective policies, procedures, and rules that are understood by employees and adhered to—safe and successful patient care goals are nearly impossible to accomplish. But employees' roles, responsibilities, status, hierarchy, and rules are only part of organizational communication. In addition, both internally with employees and externally with clients/customers/patients, as well as others stakeholders and/or potential donors, health care organizations also need to clearly communicate their mission, values, and goals.

■ MISSION, VALUES, AND GOALS

The purpose of an organization is found in its mission statement, its raison d'être. This is a communication between a company/institution/entity and its stakeholders, stockholders, customers, and vendors. Organizations, especially health care organizations, want their employees as well as their potential patients and families to recognize the way the organization views its purpose and its commitment to fulfilling that purpose vis-à-vis its organizational values and goals.

Research Exercise 8b. Go to the websites for at least two different major American organizations, one that is health care related (e.g., hospital, manufacturer, nonprofit) and one not in health care (e.g., Ford, Apple, Harvard, etc.). Research the organization's mission, values, and goals statements, often found on the home page or under "About." Once you've read these declarations, analyze how they impact your perceptions of the organization? Hypothesize if you think that was the intent of this communication? Based on these statements, is the organization a place where you would like to work and/or be a consumer; why or why not? Also, what are differences in how the health care organization portrays itself versus the non health care company? What are your thoughts on how their organizational communication affects your responses to the different entities and their products/services?

Once an organization has determined its purpose, the next logical step is for it to both decide on and then communicate the organizational goals that will be needed to fulfill its mission. These goals will help employees, as well as potential applicants and others understand the major focus of the organization's efforts. Furthermore, many institutions also communicate their values in order to inform stakeholders, stockholders, customers, and others how the organization perceives itself from an ethical perspective. The mission, goals, and values statements are important to employees because most organizations expect their members to both know them and practice them. But often, they are even more important to potential applicants. For example, if you are going to send a résumé to or interview for a position at a hospital you would be wise to carefully analyze the institution's mission, values, and goals statements to assess where your values and goals are congruent with the organization's. Based on this analysis, you would want to be sure you communicate your congruence in your cover letter and interview. In organizational communication, we know that hiring, although often described as "purposefully diverse," is still frequently biased by what has been termed "the principle of similarity." This theory suggests that we often choose our friends, lovers, and coworkers based in large part on how similar they are to us. Organizations are no different. Therefore, the more your goals and values are not "I focused," but organization-centric, the better your chance of being perceived as similar in goals and values to the organization and its members. Think about hiring from the employer's perspective, do you want to bring in a person who does not share your vision for the company? And how much more time and effort will be needed to help someone who has to be acculturated not just into a new role, but into a new coculture with its own set of goals and values? But health care organizations use more than their mission, values, and goals to communicate with stakeholders, stockholders, customers, and vendors—like most nonhealth care organizations—many rely on marketing and the media to spread their messages, as well as differentiate them from the competition.

■ MARKETING AND THE MEDIA

In 21st-century America, most organizations use a wide variety of marketing strategies and tactics to get messages about their brands, including the organization, to their consumers. Marketing includes advertising, public relations (PR), and the research efforts that support both of those, as well as various aspects of mass (TV, print, radio, Internet) and/or social media (Facebook, Instagram, Twitter, LinkedIn, etc.). Although marketing is generally not a major focus for health care providers, it is important that you recognize the role it plays in modern health care delivery. For example, many estimates suggest that the cost of numerous brand-name drugs may be driven as much, if not more, by marketing (advertising and PR) expenditures as they are by research and development (R&D) costs. Consequently, the marketing of U.S. pharmaceuticals and medical devices not only impacts patients' (direct-to-consumer [DTC] advertising and PR) and providers' (professional advertising, PR, and educational materials) perceptions of the brand, but also its cost (for patients and/or insurers). But it is not uncommon today for hospitals and other patient-focused health organizations to use marketing to help educate consumers/potential patients–providers about their employees, mission, technology, and so forth in an effort to differentiate themselves from their competition. Similarly, hospitals and other health care organizations are using social media, websites, and targeted e-mails to market themselves to potential employees and patients. The impact of marketing and media on the public's perceptions of health care, as well as on escalating health care costs, cannot be overstated. For example, if the hospital across town gets the latest robotic surgical device, a competing institution in the same town or nearby will likely feel compelled to buy a similar, or more expensive piece of technology to illustrate their value to the community. As discussed previously, this purchase may often times be more related to marketing issues than clinical ones, but in a business-model-driven health care environment, moves are made frequently for advertising and PR purposes rather than because of clinical acumen, safety, and positive outcomes. However, this increased marketing effort is generally driven by hospital administration, not health care providers.

Reflection 8.3. Think about an ad—a billboard or a newspaper, radio, TV, or Internet ad for a hospital. How does the organization's marketing of its mission, goals, and values in the ad impact your perception of the hospital? Does the fact that it is promoting certain aspects of its health care delivery make you more likely to consider it when you need hospital-based services? Or do you find it problematic in terms of your views of American health care delivery and organizational communication? Why?

_____

_____

_____

_____

_____

■ HEALTH CARE ADMINISTRATION

One significant way health organizational communication is impacted is through administration–provider communication. Although we explore the specific role and communication related to leadership in Chapter 11, it is important to recognize that administrators' verbal and nonverbal behaviors have a huge effect on the morale and functioning (or dysfunctioning) of an organization, as well as frequently being the spokespersons/face of the institution with stakeholders, customers/patients, and the public. Unlike the 20th century, when many if not most hospitals had doctors or nurses in the most executive positions, today those roles—president, chief executive officer (CEO), and so forth—are dominated by nonclinical, often business school professionals whose focus is on the functioning, income versus losses, and marketing of a hospital as much if not more than on health care delivery.

Current hospital administrators need to not only raise money and promote the institution, but adopt a business-model/competitive approach that focuses not just on the clinical expertise of the staff, but also on the technology and breadth of services available. This business mind-set can sometimes create communication obstacles for providers, who feel that patient care should be the primary, if not the only focus for everyone in the institution. In addition, the need to raise funds, assure sufficient income to meet costs, and so forth may confuse hospital employees who see the organization's stated mission, values, and goals as being more humanistic and patient centered. Therefore, it is important for providers who work at these facilities to recognize that administrators are working interdependently with clinical staff to assure the organization's safe and effective operation, as well as the need for income to further enhance the institution's health care delivery system.

Provider–administrator communication, like provider–patient and provider–provider communication is interpersonal and the more providers can work to use their verbal, nonverbal, and written communication to build relationships, share information, and seek input into decision making, the more likely it is that providers and administrators will both find the collaboration rewarding and beneficial for all, but especially for the organization. In addition, it is especially important to highlight a few key reminders for providers regarding organizational e-mail (written communication). As in all professional organizations, employees (providers) need to pay close attention to the following potential e-mail communication issues:

- For potentially problematic e-mails, do not list any names in the "To" line until you have finished editing and proofreading the e-mail, thereby avoiding accidentally sending the e-mail prematurely or to unintended recipients.

- Double or triple check that the "To" line indicates only the person(s) you intend the message for.

- Copy (cc) only people who need to know the information you are sending.

- Avoid "Reply to All" in responses to e-mails with several/numerous recipients unless it is critically important that *all* recipients need to know your reply.

- Be sure you consider that everything you send on an organization's servers (either work or private e-mail) is saved and cannot be deleted— consequently, if you do not want the CEO, your director, and/or a patient's attorney to have access to what you are e-mailing—do not send it.

- Remind yourself that whatever you put in an e-mail (text, photos, etc.) has the potential to be forwarded, sent to anyone, anywhere—so unless you want your message and/or attachments seen by unintended others, use a different communication format for sensitive communication.

- Never respond in an e-mail when you are angry—nothing good will come of it. If you receive an e-mail that upsets you, or someone says or does something, that is upsetting—try to take some time to process what happened and consider your possible communication/response options. In general, if you need to have an emotional or potentially unsettling interaction with another person it is best done face to face. Always remember that what you put in writing, especially in e-mail, will not go away—even if you delete it from your computer.

- When you need to attach a file, photo, and so forth always do it first, even before you put in the recipient's e-mail address. That way you will not forget and require the other person to have to write and ask for the attachment.

- Finally, whenever possible, consider taking a "you-" (the reader) centered approach in writing your e-mails. If you want the reader to review your message, assimilate it, and concur with you, then make the reader feel that you understand his or her needs/expectations. Use more "you," than

"I, me, my." Even "we" is more reader focused that starting every sentence with "I." Clearly, when you are taking responsibility for something, or agreeing to do something, "I" may be most appropriate, but whenever you can, try adopting a you-centered writing style and your readers are more likely to reward you with thoughtful, timely, and—perhaps more often than usual—positive responses to your requests.

Consequently, providers who are working in health care organizations as employees, consultants, contractors, and so forth need to recognize the critical role organizational communication plays in the success, not just of the institution, but in positive health care delivery outcomes. Furthermore, the recognition of how interdependent and mechanistic organizational structures, processes, and roles are—especially in health care entities—will be enormously beneficial to providers who need to work in teams to accomplish both clinical and organizational goals. The role of provider congruence with a health care organization's mission, values, and goals is also critical to the effectiveness and morale of both the provider and the rest of the organization with whom he or she works. Even though providers may have a limited role in the marketing and media aspects of a health organization's communication with stakeholders, customers/patients, and the public—it is vital that providers understand the reasons for these efforts and how they will enhance employees', providers', and patients' efforts to attain clinical and institutional goals.

Reflections (among the possible responses)

8.1. Think of two organizations (family, school, health care, religious, etc.) of which you are a member. How do you see the communication (internally and externally) being different in the two organizations, from your perspective? How does the internal communication impact your perceptions of the organization? Is one better at communicating internally (with members) than the other? If so, why?

While everyone will have very different responses to this reflection, it is important to consider how one organization, family, for example, might be perceived to have goals that are more member focused (children) and the internal communication therefore would be about how the kids needs to do certain things to enhance their mind-and-body growth, as well as their social maturity. This would be compared to a corporate organization in which the focus is on making profits and how the communication is intended to remind members (employees) of the organization's goals, the importance of keeping customers happy, and meeting deadlines, and so on. Or, if you considered a health care or religious institution, you may have perceived the organization's communication as being more collaborative and/or nurturing toward its members, but, in the case of a hospital, also its patients. However, based on your hospital experiences, you might have thought the organization was much more money/managed-care focused, not employee or patient centered, and consider the organizational communication not supportive of safe and effective health care delivery. How organizations communicate, internally especially, makes a huge difference in how much employees want to support the leaders of the institution, but also its mission, values, and goals. Employees/members, regardless of the organization, want to feel that they are similar to others, valued for their contributions, and working interdependently and collaboratively with others, including organizational leaders, to achieve common goals.

8.2. Why do you think medical, nursing, and physician assistant (PA) schools, for example, have specific, but differing, requirements to be accepted? And why do they not all teach health information from one perspective? How does this illustrate the role of organizational communication in providers' lives from earliest entry into the disciplines/professions?

As diverse cocultures in the health care culture, medical, nursing, and PA organizations are focused on not only educating and supporting their members, but also helping them assimilate into the profession/coculture. Consequently, each discipline has developed its own pedagogical approaches, curriculum, and acculturation methods to help its members adapt to their new career. For medical and osteopathic schools, there is a rigorous 4 years of study, most often postbaccalaureate, comprised of 2 primarily didactic years and 2 mostly clinically based years. However, with a doctoral degree, the provider has to get a state license to practice medicine (treat patients) and still needs to complete at least 1 year of a residency/internship program at a hospital, and pass a medical licensing exam. Nursing schools (2 and 4 years), on the other hand, have required students to focus on nursing education as the majority of their undergraduate studies. Although associate degree in nursing (ADN) programs continue to offer opportunities for students across America, a vast number of RNs are graduated each degree with a bachelor of science in nursing (BSN) degree from 4-year colleges and universities. These nursing programs differ from medical schools in diverse ways, from the degrees they confer on their graduates to the curricula they offer. In most nursing programs, the focus is on the biopsychosocial and consequently students are often introduced to clinical/patient care earlier than medical students and clinical care is continually interspersed across courses throughout their education. Upon graduation from a certified RN program, ADN and BSN students can take the national licensing exam. In order to work as an RN, a provider must pass the licensing exam. The education of PAs and APRNs is different from both RNs and MD/DOs. All of these organizational differences are intended to both continue the coculture (MD, DO, RN, etc.) and provide the knowledge and expertise students will need to function effectively and safely in their particular professions. However, from the application information materials to the verbal and nonverbal communication used in the classrooms and clinical training sites, each organization works to assure that its members are fully acculturated and understand the organization's as well as the coculture's mission, values, and goals.

8.3. Think about an ad—a billboard or a newspaper, radio, TV, or Internet ad for a hospital. How does the organization's marketing of its mission, goals, and values in the ad impact your perception of the hospital? Does the fact that it is promoting certain aspects of its health care delivery make you more likely to consider it when you need hospital-based services? Or do you find it problematic in terms of your views of American health care delivery and organizational communication? Why?

Generally speaking, health care organizations use advertising, regardless of the format, just like non health care organizations. The goal of advertising is to promote a brand, provide information about it, and offer some call to action (purchase, promote, inquire, etc.). The question for most health care advertising is do we highlight our people, services, technologies, and so on? How a health care organization answers that question is often based on its mission, values, and goals, but may also be driven by a marketing analysis that perceives a competitive message more important than a patient- or provider-centric one. However, your responses to a health care organization's advertising is usually a good indicator of your congruence—from an employee or patient perspective—with the organization's communication of its mission, values, and goals. Because advertising is expensive and usually involves a significant amount of critical thinking, reflection, and analysis, the verbal and nonverbal messages are generally what the organization wants viewers/readers to know about itself and its health care delivery services.

Skills Exercise

Think of an organization you belong to (family, school, religious, professional, etc.) and select what aspects of the chosen organization's purpose, goals, and values you think would be important for a person to know in order to perceive the organization positively. Based on that analysis, create a script for yourself to use in communicating to a friend, colleague, or peer who is unfamiliar (not a part of) with the organization you are discussing. Share your information about the organization with the other interactant. Use feedback to assess his or her understanding and further explain, or, if clear, ask what the other person thinks about such an organization? Would he or she want to work there, be a customer, or a member in some way? How does assessing an organization and communicating about it help you understand the way organizational communication, if done effectively, can benefit both the institution and its members/employees, stakeholders, customers, and so forth?

Video Discussion Exercise

Analyze the video

- *Lorenzo's Oil* (1992)

Interactive Simulation Exercise

Pagano, M. (2015). *Communication case studies for health care professionals: An applied approach* (2nd ed.). New York, NY: Springer Publishing Company.

- Chapter 30, "How Safe are Generics?" (pp. 293–300)
- Chapter 38, "Health Insurance Portability and Accountability Act (HIPAA)" (pp. 367–374)
- Chapter 42, "What's an Interdisciplinary Meeting?" (pp. 399–406)

Health Care Issues in the Media

Hospitals hiring doctors
http://health.usnews.com/health-news/hospital-of-tomorrow/articles/2015/10/07/whistleblower-doctor-warns-about-hospitals-hiring-physicians

Health Communication Outcomes

Health care organizational communication impacts all areas of health care delivery in America. Whether it is a hospital, hospice, pharmaceutical or medical device manufacturer, or health insurance company—all are organized by and require effective internal and external communication to succeed. In health organizations, there are numerous communication demands; however, the most common is interpersonal communication—for providers and patients, providers and providers, as well as providers and administrators. However, provider–provider communication frequently needs to be team focused, rather than dyadic, and, in order to share information, it is often necessary for providers to be public speakers, especially at hospital grand rounds conferences or in various continuing-education and training contexts. Furthermore, administrators and some providers may also be expected to use mass communication and educate the stakeholders, customers/patients and families, as well as the general public about the organization and its health care delivery services. These mass-media formats can include print, TV, Internet, and/or radio, as well as various social media possibilities. Regardless of to whom or how an organization's message is delivered—to be most effective the institution needs to not only have a clear and consistent mission, goals, and values statements, but communicate them in all forms of internal and external organizational messages. Sharing the organization's culture with external sources is best managed using carefully assessed and developed advertising, PR, and media marketing campaigns. Finally, the evolving role of senior administrators in hospitals and other health care organizations highlights the potential communication challenges for providers who feel that these institutions should be more patient focused rather than business focused. Consequently, providers need to strive to enhance their interpersonal relationships with administrators vis-à-vis their effective verbal and nonverbal interpersonal/organizational communication.

■ BIBLIOGRAPHY

Apker, J. (2012). *Communication in health organizations*. Cambridge, MA: Polity Press.

Borkowski, N. (2016). Organizational behavior in health care. In *Part IV, intrapersonal and interpersonal issues* (3rd ed., pp. 251–329). Burlington, MA: Jones & Bartlett.

Borkowski, N., & Deckard, G. (Eds.). (2014). Case studies in organizational behavior and theory for health care. In *Case seventeen: Working toward collaborative care* (pp. 113–136). Sudbury, MA: Jones & Bartlett.

Kenney, C. (2010). A journey to Japan. In *Transforming healthcare: Virginia Mason Medical Center's pursuit of the perfect patient experience* (pp. 13–32). New York, NY: Taylor & Francis.

Mick, S., & Wyttenbach, M. (Eds.). (2003). Understanding health care markets. In *Advances in health care organization theory* (pp. 99–141). San Francisco, CA: Jossey-Bass.

O'Shea, E., Pagano, M., Campbell, S., & Caso, G. (2013). A descriptive analysis of nursing student communication behaviors. *Clinical Simulation in Nursing, 9*(1), e5–e12. doi:10.1016/j.ecns.2011.05.013

Shi, L., & Singh, D. (2015). Delivering health care in America: A systems approach. In *Inpatient facilities and services* (6th ed., pp. 291–335). Burlington, MA: Jones & Bartlett.

Shockley-Zalabak, P. (2015). Fundamentals of organizational communication: Knowledge, sensitivity, skills, values. In *Communication implications of major organizational theories* (9th ed., pp. 70–83). Boston, MA: Pearson.

The Joint Commission. (2016). *Hospital accreditation*. Retrieved from http://www.jointcommission.org/accreditation/hospitals.aspx

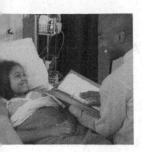

CHAPTER 9

Team Communication

For the purpose of this text, we are going to use the following as working definitions:

- *Clinical simulation:* Health care providers (students and/or professionals) role-playing scripted scenarios to enhance clinical care, health communication, and reduce provider stress; may include a student/professional, or paid actors or can be done with a computerized mannequin

- *Communication climate:* The atmosphere, environment, and/or conditions that impact small-group/team communication; can be positive, neutral, or negative

- *Norms:* Rules or standards groups/teams use to communicate what behaviors are acceptable, expected, and/or unacceptable

- *Small-group/team communication:* Three to 20 individuals working together interdependently to accomplish common goals; 13 is thought to be the ideal number for a small group/team

- *Social exchange theory:* Explains group/team behavior in terms of positives and negative relationships and rewards

- *Symbolic convergence theory:* Posits that communication helps inform and construct a group/team's culture as well its communication behaviors and decision making

- *Systems theory:* Describes group/team as a system that uses information from a variety of sources, internal and external, to process, analyze, and act on that information in order to attain a desired outcome or goal

- *Team climate:* The environment/feeling that members create and promote vis-à-vis their communication behaviors (can be positive/supportive or negative/defensive)

■ TEAM COMMUNICATION IN HOSPITALS/ HEALTH CARE

As we have previously discussed, especially in hospitals and acute care facilities, 21st-century American health care is much more team focused than individualized. It should be noted that for the purpose of this book, the term *team communication* is used, but in reality, that term is readily exchangeable with *small-group communication*. Also, although most organizations today are team oriented, health care delivery systems, especially hospitals, have very diverse members who are patient-centered stakeholders (employees, contractors, consultants, etc.) and may not all be employed members of the same organization (but functioning as such). For example, it is not uncommon in many emergency departments (EDs) today for the physicians, physician assistants, and advanced practice nurses to not be hospital employees, but rather contracted labor from an emergency medicine group (e.g., Emergency Medicine Physicians [EMP] in Canton, Ohio). Similarly, because EMP, like all contractors, may not be able to find enough ED providers in a particular city to staff a particular contracted hospital, EMP may use "fire fighters," ED providers from other cities who are sent to a particular hospital for protracted periods of time (locum tenens), usually weeks or months. Therefore, the critically important ED team of MD/DO (doctor of osteopathy), RN, physician assistant (PA), advanced practice registered nurse (APRN), and technicians who are required for effective emergency care often may be comprised of members who are not employed by the same institution. In addition, because of staffing needs (24/7/365), hospital teams, ED and others, frequently include members who are interchangeable (recall our discussion of hiring/staffing, standardized and replaceable members for organizational success), for example, the scrub nurse for a hip replacement in the morning will almost certainly be different for the same procedure, even the same surgeon that night. This need for teams and interdependent behaviors that coalesce into successful outcomes is a key element of differentiation between team membership in hospital-styled institutions and other nonhospital-type organizations.

Reflection 9.1. Think about a nonhospital team/group you have been or are a member of. What would be the impact on the team's goals if tomorrow someone with the same skills suddenly replaced one member? And then 2 days later, the original member returns, but now a different member is replaced? How would you expect these changes to impact the team's process, production, communication, time management, and outcomes? Why?

As you can see, the use of teams in hospitals (and hospital-like entities, hospices, rehabilitation centers, long-term care facilities, etc.) is both critical to the organization's goals, but also to safe and effective patient care. In most nonhospital-like organizations (corporate, for profit, nonprofit, etc.), teams are created based on the team's role/goals, and careful attention is paid to the individual potential contributions to the team's efforts by specific employees. In hospitals, teams are used to maximize health care delivery, provide "checks and balances" in the assessment of decisions, plans, and behaviors/actions. For example, in a typical acute-care hospital there are likely surgical, medical, obstetrics, and pediatrics units that care for inpatients 24/7/365. In many hospitals today, such a unit would utilize a team approach to patient care that at the very least would include one or more of the following members:

- RNs (usually discipline specific, medicine vs. surgery, etc.)
- MD/DOs (almost always discipline specific, board certified in surgery vs. pediatrics), patient's private doctor versus hospitalist
- Licensed practical nurses (LPNs; nurses who work under the supervision of RNs and are usually less discipline specific)
- PAs or APRNs (usually discipline specific, but may be more generalist than MD/DO; work under the supervision of the private, or hospitalist, MD/DO)
- Residents (MD/DO, discipline specific, but of varying years of experience, usually 1–5 years post-MD/DO degree)
- Students (RN, APRN, PA, at various stages of their education/clinical training and available for different periods of time, from 1 day a week or less, to an entire 6–8 weeks)
- Technicians/nursing assistants (may be unit specific or may float between units/disciplines as needed)

As you can quickly see, a team for one unit of a hospital can have anywhere from seven to 10 or more team members, especially if there are private doctors on the team, students, and so forth. But again, the distinction here is that the makeup of that team—from a professional perspective—may be constant, one of each from the previous list, but the individual—physician, RN, PA, resident, and so forth—will likely change not just daily, but two or three times per day (depending on whether staffing is on 8- or 12-hour shifts). Consequently, if you worked at Ford or Apple, or any other major organization in America and you were placed on a team, in all likelihood the makeup of that team would be static because stability is expected to benefit from the predictability of the team individually and collectively. And, in many organizations, the specific members of teams are maintained for months, if not years. However, in health care there is hardly a portion of a day that goes by without the health care team having different individuals rotate through. Therefore, the dialectical tension between the need to work together but with a variety of regularly changing team members, underlies the critical importance of effective interpersonal and team communication.

The use of teams in hospitals is both vital to successful health care delivery as well as to overall organizational goal attainment. Teams help health care organizations accomplish numerous goals by (a) increasing diverse input into analysis and decision making; (b) offering interdisciplinary/interprofessional approaches; and (c) providing more opportunities for explorations of ideas, assessments, interventions, and plans. This modern approach to health care delivery is far different than the physician-centric model that was the norm for thousands of years. From ancient Egypt to the late 20th century, health care delivery was primarily the purview of physicians who diagnosed and treated patients. However, this physician-focused method did not utilize a team approach to patient care, but frequently relied on nonphysicians (usually nurses) to dutifully carry out the physician's orders/instructions/prescriptions. But with the introduction of midlevel providers (certified registered nurse anesthetists [CRNA], PAs, APRNs, etc.), evolving RN roles, economic considerations, and managed care—hospitals and health care providers have reoriented their approaches to patient care to follow a more collaborative, diverse, and inclusive team model.

With the ever-increasing quantities of wellness/illness/injury knowledge, technology development, treatment options, and health care costs it is critical for hospitals to find an organizational communication approach to patient care that can adapt quickly and effectively. Consequently, interprofessional teams have evolved as the primary method most institutions use to accomplish clinical/patient goals, enhance health care delivery, and overcome risks. Unlike nonhospital organizations, hospitals' health care goals and patient needs/expectations require teams to be constantly working to assess and resolve the daily patient–provider task, problem, and/or solution issues that exist 24/7/365 in modern hospitals. And, unlike many organizations that are not even open 24/7/365, hospitals need teams (of administrators and providers) to develop policies and procedures for the daily care of patients, but also regarding:

- How to handle a catastrophic event with dozens or more injured
- Outbreaks of rare contagious diseases
- Shortening wait times in the ED
- Increasing the arrival time of the code team at a dying patient's bedside

Therefore, the value of patient care teams to the organization's success and goal attainment is only overshadowed by the importance of countless teams' efforts in almost every aspect of a hospital's daily health care delivery process. In order for hospitals to utilize their staff and facilities most effectively they must rely on diverse health care providers, each with his or her professional input, analysis, and critical thinking, contributing to teams that often have interchangeable members from the same profession.

This consistent, dialectical tension between needing a particular discipline represented on a team, but not being able to control which professional is working on the team on any given day is truly unique to hospital-like institutions. Therefore, it should not be surprising to recognize the need for effective interpersonal and team communication in order to accomplish a hospital team's goals and objectives—in spite of the lack of individual predictability of members.

Let's examine just one potential problem for a health care team that is constructed with specific professional members (physician, nurse, resident, midlevel provider, etc.), but on any given day (or at any given meeting time) the members could be all the same as previously, or they could all be completely different. For example, Sara is Mr. Jones's surgeon, she makes rounds (sees her patients) with her PA, Molly; Mr. Jones's 7:00 a.m. to 3:00 p.m. RN, Jim; the surgical residents, Frank, Mary, and Miles; and two nursing students, Hillary and Betty. These eight providers go to the patient's bedside, talk and/or listen to the conversation with the patient, observe the dressing change, and discuss the treatment plan for the day. At 8:00 p.m., the same day, Cathy is the RN caring for Mr. Jones who has spiked an oral temperature of 101.6°F and is complaining of increased pain around his wound. Cathy did not see the patient at morning rounds, or talk with any of the team—except Jim at shift change. Jim provided his usual hand off—situation, background, assessment, and recommendation (SBAR)—for each of the patients he was turning over to Cathy. Therefore, Cathy knew from Mr. Jones's SBAR, as well as her review of his electronic medical record (EMR), that he did not complain of pain, or have a fever earlier in the day. She also knows that although there is an order for an antipyretic, acetaminophen (to lower his temperature), fever and pain in a postoperative patient are often indicative of more serious wound or lung infections that need to be assessed. Consequently, Cathy gets the patient's prescribed medication, but also telephones Molly, Dr. Jones's PA, as well as Henry, the surgical resident on duty. Molly asks Cathy to have Henry call her after he examines the patient. Molly tells Cathy that although she is on call that night, Dr. Watt is covering for Dr. Jones and Molly will make Dr. Watt aware of the situation as soon as she hears back from Henry, but in the meantime to please call if Mr. Jones gets worse, if Cathy has any questions, or Henry cannot come see the patient soon.

This example illustrates just one aspect of the onerous nature of 21st-century health care in America. Although teams are used to improve patient care and reduce risks, the members of these teams cannot function 24/7/365. Therefore, hospital teams not only have to work as cohesive, collaborative units, but do so with interchangeable members whose professional education and experiences are similar—even though their identities and backgrounds are clearly disparate. Originally, there are eight providers from diverse professions who are functioning as a task-oriented, problem-solving, and decision-making team. However, 12 hours later, none of the original eight team members are in the hospital, let alone available to meet and assess the patient's problem and derive a solution.

But because of the communication, education, and team processes utilized in hospitals and hospital-like facilities, the different team members at 8:00 p.m. functioned in many ways like the earlier team. First, Cathy used the information from her peer, Jim, to understand the patient's condition, but she also used the morning team's assessment and plan from the EMR. Second, when Mr. Jones's health changed, based on the data Cathy was given (verbally and in writing, as well as her own assessment of the patient), she fulfilled her team role and responsibilities by first providing medication that was ordered. Third, she also notified the appropriate (based on the team structure and vertical hierarchy) team members of the change in the patient's signs (fever) and symptoms (peri-wound pain). This new, but consistent health care team must now focus on problem solving with certain members, surgical resident, RN, PA, and eventually the oncall surgeon to work collaboratively and interdependently to assess the problem, identify the cause, and find the most effective solution. In order for this to occur, Cathy needs to both assess the patient as well as communicate with Henry, the surgical resident. Once Henry has assimilated Cathy's information, with his own patient assessment, he will need to communicate that by phone to Molly. Based on Cathy and Henry's findings and Henry's recommendations, Molly will need to determine if there is a need for her to examine the patient, order further tests, or contact Dr. Watt. At every stage of this problem-solving process information is expanded vis-à-vis input from multiple sources with diverse health education and experiences all contributing to the analysis and decision making. As current or future health care providers/professionals, you need to understand how these teams function, what makes one team more effective than another, and how to address conflict and/or communication problems. Furthermore, although the previous examples are hospital/hospital-like institution specific, please recognize that private practice offices, public/community health clinics, stand-alone urgent care facilities, and so forth all use team communication to accomplish their organizational and patient care goals.

■ A SYSTEMS APPROACH

Although there are a number of small-group/team communication theories, we are going to focus on systems theory. Clearly, health care team communication can be viewed using a variety of theoretical lenses, including social exchange theory and symbolic convergence theory, as well as others (structuration, functional, etc.). However, for the purposes of this text a systems approach seems to be the most appropriate (and some would argue the most common approach regardless of organizational type, goals, etc.). Systems theory views team communication as a group of subsystems, with each member (subsystem) of the team providing different skills, knowledge, expertise, and input to help attain team/organizational goals. As you can tell, systems theory is about skilled individuals, in our case, health professionals working together to accomplish tasks, solve problems, make decisions, and so forth. For health care teams, this interprofessional approach heightens the interdependent possibilities for exploring diverse viewpoints, opportunities, analyses, and solutions/plans. Furthermore, a systems-theory approach would suggest that the more health care teams function interdependently to gather information (from the patient, objective data [vital signs, labs/tests, procedures], other providers, scholarly literature, etc.) and analyze it from diverse professional perspectives, the more likely they will be to effectively address problems, develop (and when necessary revise) solutions/treatment plans, and enhance decision making with the patient. However, successful outcomes/goal attainments are dependent on a number of key communication factors related to team development: roles, norms, status, and relationships.

■ TEAM DEVELOPMENT

As previously noted, health care teams are unique in many ways; however, members of such teams are generally first hired related to their profession, certification licensures, and so forth. In fact, most hospital hiring is still done in professions—independent of the interdisciplinary team structure that most hospital providers are expected to work in. Consequently, nurses are hired by nurses, physicians and physician assistants by physicians, and so forth. In some non health care organizations in which a person is being hired to function primarily as part of a team, that applicant likely would be interviewed and assessed by one or more members of the team he or she would be working with, as well as his or her department/unit/organization manager/supervisor.

Reflection 9.2. Can you recall a team you were a member of—sports, academic, or professional—how did you work interdependently to accomplish the team's goals? What made that team different from others that were not as successful?

_____

_____

_____

_____

_____

Because of the independent nature of 21st-century health care regarding professional identity, hospital teams are often developed—not through a primary team focus (interprofessional)—but intraprofessionally, with professional peers making the hiring decisions. However, soon after a hospital provider is hired, he or she is expected to work in a number of intra- and interprofessional teams. For example, physicians (as well as residents) are expected to work with other MDs to assure coverage/staffing, policy and procedural regulations, effective patient care, as well as peer review in conflict situations. This same approach is true in nursing. However, PAs—who by law must be supervised by physicians—are viewed as part of the physician intraprofessional team, not nursing. APRNs may be hired under either the nursing or physician intraprofessional team. Consequently, the members of countless health care teams seldom have any relationship with the other providers in their interprofessional team until they meet as part of their work experience. Therefore, if you go to work for a hospital, intraprofessional peers who are not part of your interprofessional teams will likely hire you.

If you recall our previous examples, the patient had a specific physician; however, that physician may have someone else covering for him/her at night, on weekends, vacations, or holidays. Similarly, the patient will likely receive care from a minimum of two different nurses each day, but they can be different from one day to the next. This unique team approach, which does not include specific members but rather interchangeable profession-dependent individuals, creates a major need for effective team communication and role identity.

■ ROLES

Health care roles, especially in hospitals, are clearly defined, therefore, certain members can order treatments, others carry out those orders, some members can work in surgery, or labor and delivery, and so forth; these roles are generally codified vis-à-vis a member's academic degree and state licensure. Consequently, an RN's role is related to but distinct from a PA, MD, certified nursing assistant (CNA), and so forth. The benefit for unique health care teams—in some situations teams are formed and dissolved on a daily basis—is that there is no time spent questioning a member's role. In health care generally provider's roles are clearly defined, regulated, and communicated. Therefore, the RN who starts a shift at 7:00 a.m. expects the intraprofessional team to be other RNs who are both educated and licensed as he or she is. Similarly, the RN expects the members of the interprofessional teams to be comprised of providers who have been assigned, like herself or himself, to the care of a particular patient. Therefore, the team may be patient centered and the RN may very well have a different team for each of her patients on any given day. This same reality is true for the other professional members of a hospital team. The obstetrician–physician who has a patient in labor may have worked with some of the RNs who are caring for the patient, but he or she may not know the CRNA, or the scrub nurse, neonatal APRN, and so forth if a caesarean section (c-section) is required.

The critical importance of having clearly identifiable and highly codifed roles is one of the major reasons why health care teams are so effective. The team members generally assume each other's credibility and capability, based on a person's academic degree, title, and license. However, successful teamwork, goal attainment, and/or patient outcomes do not happen automatically based on members' roles. Teams need to collaborate, fully participate, and effectively communicate and that doesn't just rely on roles, but also on clearly understood team norms.

Reflection 9.3. How do you think the clarity of role distinctions in health care teams might enhance and/or diminish effective interprofessional communication? Why?

_____

_____

_____

_____

_____

■ NORMS

Teams need norms in order to assure that everyone understands, not just his or her professional, but intrateam goals. For example, one health care team norm might be that no one uses his or her status to insult or demean anyone on the team. A typical norm, as we have seen in prior examples, is that the team in a hospital unit understands that its members will all meet—regardless of who the individuals are, to review the patient's progress, address any issues, and work with the patient to determine a plan for next steps. Consequently, for one team, the norm might be to "make rounds" at 6:30 a.m., whereas a different team might do its patient visits starting at 7:00 a.m. Other norms may be focused on who starts the presentation, or who examines the patient first, and so forth. These norms are not static and my change based on members or context within an interprofessional team, but almost surely will have some variances across all intra- and interprofessional teams. Therefore, it would be expected that norms for an inter- and intraprofessional team would be different when making rounds than in surgery, or the delivery room, and so forth. Clearly, providers need to recognize that like roles, norms need to be communicated and understood, but unlike roles, norms are context and intra- and/or interprofessional team dependent. However, just as norms are critical for effective team communication, so too is understanding how status differences impact team communication.

Reflection 9.4. Can you recall some norms, stated or understood, for a team you were a member of? How did these norms aid or detract from effective communication and/or goal attainment? Why?

_____

_____

_____

_____

_____

■ STATUS

In health care organizations, especially hospitals, status is frequently determined and/or perceived based on members' titles: CEO, chief nursing officer (CNO), director, manager, and so forth for administrators and by academic degrees/licenses: MD/DO, RN, APRN, PA, and so forth for providers/clinicians. And even though providers may have the same degree, board certification, and license, there are often status distinctions within intraprofessional teams. For example, some members may have higher status among peers based on research, publications, professional reputation, clinical skills, and so forth. However, status can have even more of a profound impact on interprofessional teams and their communication behaviors.

Because for centuries health care has afforded higher status to physicians than other health care providers—especially when it came to patient care decision making, it is only recently that status among interprofessional team members has been questioned and/or considered. However, we know a number of important realities about the role of status in group/team communication (regardless of the organization—health care related or not), including:

1. Just as in patient–provider communication, the interprofessional team members with higher status can be expected to speak more than those with lower status.

2. High-status interprofessional members can be expected to communicate more intraprofessionally, than interprofessionally (e.g., MDs/DOs and residents, or RNs and APRNs).

3. Interprofessional members who perceive their status to be lower than other members generally communicate more positively to higher status teammates than to their equals or lower status members.

4. Team members may focus on and/or more frequently accept high-status members' suggestions over lower status members' analyses and recommendations.

As you can see there are some very serious status consequences for interprofessional health care teams unless they recognize the risks early and discuss how they can both address the status realities and minimize the potential information sharing, tasks, and/or decision-making difficulties related to them.

Reflection 9.5. Have you worked in a group/team in which one or more members had a higher status than you? If so, how did it impact your group/ team communication? If not, what are your views of the issues listed previously in terms of status differences?

_____

_____

_____

_____

_____

Therefore, based on the possible impact of status differences in interprofessional health care teams, there needs to be a communication strategy for members to use to avoid, or at least limit, these negative effects. If members recognize how higher status individuals tend to dominate conversations, then the team might want to have an appointed discussion leader who does not have the highest status and who is empowered to assure equal input in discussions. For example, an interdisciplinary hospice team might use an RN, social worker, or chaplain to lead its meetings and while needing and encouraging input from physicians, nurses, and others, the discussion leader would make every effort to give equal time and opportunity to all professionals on the team. Similarly, the team might agree on a norm that discourages "sidebar" conversations intra- and interprofessionally in order to minimize both the distractions, but also to limit similar-status members communicating with each other instead of with the team. Furthermore, teams might want to try to prevent other status issues by agreeing on norms that discourage members from using "group think" communication and agreeing to what others have proposed related to status differences. Similarly, encourage members, regardless of status, to be honest with the team when communicating their viewpoints. It will not serve the interprofessional team well if lower status members are not communicating their perspectives with everyone. Separate conversations with perceived equal and/or lower status team members during which different views are expressed than those stated with higher status teammates can only serve to minimize the diversity of input into the team's decision making, but also negatively impact the team's dynamics and culture by lowering morale. Interprofessional teams need to both understand and address the issues related to roles, norms, and status if they are to develop trusting relationships and effective interprofessional team communication.

■ RELATIONSHIPS

In order to enhance interprofessional health care teams, it is important to focus on interpersonal communication. Even though teams function as a collective, at their core, most teams are greatly impacted by interpersonal communication in order for members to develop professional interpersonal relationships. And as we have discussed previously, Americans often trust and prefer to work with others who are similar to themselves. The same can be expected in health care teams; however, by their very nature, these interprofessional teams are diverse in a number of key areas:

- Profession
- Health care experience
- Age
- Sex
- Status

Consequently, interprofessional health care teams must rely on members' efforts to develop professional relationships that will help them overcome their differences, increase trust, and use that diversity to enhance group outcomes. In fact, the diverse nature as well as interchangeable aspect of interprofessional health care teams affords them great opportunities. For example, when providers work independently, an MD/DO/PA/APRN sees a patient in the hospital, writes orders and moves on to the next patient, procedure, office, and so forth. Then the RN is expected to read the orders and carry them out, often with little or no input or discussion about the patient's history since the last time the patient was seen by the provider writing the orders. In addition, the RN does not generally have any explanation for why one treatment plan is being used versus another and no easy way to communicate issues that the RN wants to discuss. Therefore, the patient's care and decision making are being negatively impacted by the lack of information sharing and diverse input. Also, the lack of face-to-face communication and/or information sharing among various professionals who are caring for the patient, further risks miscommunication and/or missing data. Going back 20 years or more, hospital health care roles were very rigid and resulted in a more linear and authoritarian approach to communication and decision making. In that era, an MD independently did "X," and RNs and other non-MDs followed his or her orders/decisions. However, it has been demonstrated through health care risk management, quality control, and organizational communication that everyone benefits from a diverse interprofessional team approach to information exchanges and patient care. Although it is true that the MD/DO is ultimately responsible for the decisions and hospital orders—that legal reality can be enhanced by interprofessional health care teams that use interpersonal communication to develop trusting relationships and minimize the authoritarian nature of decision making and encourage a much more collaborative, participative team approach that benefits from the team members' diversity, input, and critical thinking. However, health care team members have specific administrative and/or clinical roles, but in addition, teams generally have members who take on specific team roles.

■ TEAM ROLES

Just as it is important for team members to understand each other's professional roles, it is very helpful to recognize the various team roles that members may assume. In fact, Benne and Sheats (1948) created a list of possible team roles that members may utilize, including:

- Aggressor
- Blocker
- Recognition seeker
- Joker
- Dominator

These various team roles are generally recognizable to anyone who has been a part of any type of team, from our families, to sports teams, to health care teams. It is important for interprofessional teams to understand that in addition to, or in some cases related to, a member's clinical or administrative role, he or she may use the role to impact team dynamics and communication exchanges. As you know from your experiences in groups/teams, these roles can be beneficial to the overall goals of the members. However, some of these roles can create trust and relationship development problems within the team. Therefore, interprofessional health care teams have to recognize when members are using one of these roles in an effort to thwart interaction, information sharing, collaboration, and/or participation. For example, a joker can be a helpful role in a team—as long as the member is not using humor as a way to block discussions. However, once an individual member assumes one of these roles, the team must be willing to address the issue of how it impacts, positively or negatively, the team's tasks, goals, and dynamics. This ability to identify potential team problems is critically important, but also must be viewed in the context of positive versus negative team conflict.

Reflection 9.6. Recall one of the groups/teams you are/have been a member of (family, team, school, professional) and reflect on how a member assumed one of the roles and communicated based on that. How did his or her role/behaviors impact the group's/team's work and your perception of the group/team?

_____

_____

_____

_____

_____

■ MANAGING CONFLICT

First and foremost, it is important to recognize that conflict, in and of itself, is not a bad thing. Conflict is basically a disagreement, but in terms of communication and decision making, disagreements are opportunities to explore other ideas, approaches, and viewpoints. One of the benefits of interprofessional health care teams that we have been discussing is the importance of members' diversity. However, the benefits of members' uniqueness (professional, role, age, etc.) lies in their abilities to provide a variety of different contributions to whatever topic, role, task, or goal the team is working on. As mentioned previously, team think is the opposite of conflict. Team think occurs when members just agree with whatever is being proposed, rather than offering conflicting views, ideas, or alternatives. Consider a team in which everyone just agrees with one member's recommendations (team think) without debate and consideration of other options—consequently, the possibilities that the unspoken, unconsidered, and unanalyzed alternatives might have resulted in a better outcome are unknown. Also, recognize that without conflict, teams would really have nothing to discuss and no real purpose. However, although team conflict is both necessary and positive for exploring diverse options for completing tasks, addressing/solving problems, and accomplishing goals, some forms of team conflict can be destructive and inhibit effective interprofessional health care team communication and outcomes.

Negative conflicts in teams can result from a variety of social behaviors. For example, some members of a team may have different viewpoints than others, biases or perceptions about various issues and be unwilling to change. Not surprisingly, individual personalities can lead to problematic differences in opinions, or worse, an unwillingness to share information and communicate openly with other team members. Also knowledge differences, not just related to health education but to what is shared among members, can lead to problematic team conflict. Similarly, differences in members' cultures and cocultures, as well as status differences (perceived and real) can lead to disagreements and obstacles to effective interprofessional team communication. It is important to also note that conflicts can be directed at people (a member or members), or at tasks (ideas, decisions, problem solving, etc.), or both. Team members need to identify the most effective communication approach to overcoming negative/unproductive conflict.

One of the ways to overcome conflict is to use effective interpersonal communication and try to both understand the other person's views and, if possible, why he or she holds them. Although it may be helpful to try and persuade the person to consider a different approach to the disagreement, if that does not work, members can try to find a compromise that can result in a win–win–win for involved members, but also for the entire team. However, teams should be very careful to not allow a conflict, regardless of its origin, to dissolve into a personal attack on a member, or communication behaviors that can be perceived as emotionally aggressive and/or hostile. To minimize negative/unproductive conflict and maximize diverse inputs/productive conflict, teams need to develop a supportive climate.

A supportive team climate is an environment in which members feel comfortable sharing information, voicing concerns and/or differing viewpoints. Tandy (1992) pointed out that the more supportive the team climate the more likely it will reduce stress and burnout for members and increase team productivity. Furthermore, a supportive climate is enhanced not just by the verbal messages that members communicate, but also through their nonverbal cues (proxemics, kinesics, volume, tone, etc.). Also, teams generally respond positively when members think that they share some common feelings for one another. Therefore, empathic messages and listening communicate a caring attitude to teammates. Not surprising, the more equality and openness to others' ideas, concerns, and communication team members can demonstrate, the more supportive the team climate will be perceived. Finally, in order to avoid a defensive/unproductive team climate, members need to try and avoid verbal and nonverbal behaviors that can be perceived by others as evaluating, controlling, uncaring, or superior. It is especially important to try to discourage members from taking rigid and egocentric approaches to information sharing, problem solving, and/or decision making—all of which negatively impact both the team climate and the opportunity to encourage diverse input and exploration. Interprofessional health care teams by their very nature have a number of obstacles to overcome related to roles, norms, status, and organizational structure. However, by using effective team communication to encourage information sharing, diverse viewpoints, and a supportive climate, interprofessional health care teams can be extremely productive, successful, and beneficial in attaining both the team and organization's goals as well as ensuring the most effective patient care possible.

Reflections (among the possible responses)

9.1. Think about a nonhospital team/group you have been or are a member of. What would be the impact on the team's goals if tomorrow someone with the same skills suddenly replaced one member? And then 2 days later, the original member returns, but now a different member is replaced? How would you expect these changes to impact the team's process, production, communication, time management, and outcomes? Why?

Generally, most teams/groups have members who are consistent for the most part. Think of a professional sports team, for example, most of them perform much better and attain their goals the more they can keep the makeup of the team constant. Clearly, members may have to move in and out for injuries or unexpected life events, but the more frequent the change in personnel, the less likely the team will function at its ultimate capacity and attain both its and the organization's goals—winning a championship for a professional sports team. Some of the reasons why the evolving membership negatively impacts team performance is related not just to the specific skills, knowledge, and athleticism of the individuals (in or out), but also to the changes in nonverbal and verbal interpersonal and team communication among the teammates. This notion of constancy and its impact on team outcomes makes the amazing work of health care interprofessional teams—with the constant change in specific members coupled with frequent goal attainment—seem very impressive, but also important to be very aware of as team members.

9.2. Can you recall a team you were a member of—sports, academic, or professional— how did you work interdependently to accomplish the team's goals? What made that team different from others that were not as successful?

Regardless of the team—sports, academic, or professional—in all likelihood you brought your individual skills, talents, and knowledge to your role and, when combined interpersonally with the other members of the team, the members'/team's goals were attained. In order to be successful it is critical for a team to have the most effective combination of individuals, roles, and skills needed, but it is just as important to have those members not just function independently, but collaboratively. In order to do that most effectively, positive and productive team climate and communication that encourages participation, diversity, and supportive behaviors are required.

9.3. How do you think the clarity of role distinctions in health care teams might enhance and/or diminish effective interprofessional communication? Why?

In health care, clinical roles are clearly delineated by academic degree, certification, licensure, and so forth. Whether a provider is an MD/DO, RN, APRN, PA, his or her role is very obvious to all members of the hospital or other health care organization. Therefore, health care teams are generally comprised based on cocultures—intraprofessional teams (physicians, or nurses, or PAs), as well as on interprofessional teams (MD/DO, RN, PA, APRN, resident, etc.). The clearly designated roles/professions of the various members alleviate any questions regarding clinical roles. However, the team roles and whether status, power, or diversity will lead to a supportive or defensive team climate must be constantly assessed, as well as the impact of the interchangeable nature of specific individuals on the culture of interprofessional health care teams.

9.4. Can you recall some norms, stated or understood, for a team you were a member of? How did these norms aid or detract from effective communication and/or goal attainment? Why?

Teams all have norms, some are clearly communicated: you should be here by 8:00 a.m. Or you are expected to be ready to present your patient when the team enters the room. However, others may not be communicated but are understood—if you are a member of a sports team you need to be dedicated and perform to your maximum potential. Similarly, in health care interprofessional teams, some of the norms could be related to who takes notes, or who gathers the patients' lab values, vital signs, and so forth. Norms are critically important to the effective communication and functioning of interprofessional teams. Part of each team member's responsibility is to learn the team's norms and share them with new members in order to assure expected behaviors and maximum information sharing and time management.

9.5. Have you worked in a group/team in which one or more members had a higher status than you? If so, how did it impact your group/team communication? If not, what are your views of the issues listed previously in terms of status differences?

It is not uncommon, especially in families and professional groups/teams, for members to have different levels of status. For example, parents in a family group/team usually have a higher status than their children, and, based on birth order, siblings often have lower status if they are not the oldest, and so forth. On sports teams, coaches and/or captains often have perceived higher status than other members. In health care teams, doctors often have higher status, followed by nurses and midlevel providers. However, in order for teams to function most effectively, members need to feel that status differences should not impact tasks, information sharing, idea generation, problem solving, and/or decision-making goals. Although status in health care is a long-standing reality, the current effort to increase diversity and interprofessional collaboration and participation seeks to minimize the impact of status on team communication and increase the value of diverse input and analyses in patient care.

9.6. Recall one of the groups/teams you are/have been a member of (family, team, school, professional) and reflect on how a member assumed one of the roles and communicated based on that. How did his or her role/behaviors impact the group's/team's work and your perception of the group/team?

Many teams/groups have members who choose to take on a team role, for example, there may be a "blocker" in a group/team you have been a member of. This person perceives his or her role as constantly being the so-called "devil's advocate" and stubbornly disagrees with most, if not all suggestions, ideas, and so forth; at times the blocker can appear to be creating conflict for no apparent reason—other than to be negative and an obstructionist. Clearly, members who assume roles that detract from effective team communication can make it very difficult to complete tasks, solve problems, make decisions, and attain goals. Consequently, teams must be very cognizant of how members are communicating/behaving and work together to try and discourage members from assuming team roles that will be detrimental to effective communication and a supportive team climate.

Skills Exercise

In a team that you are active in, family, school, work, health care, and so forth, ask as many individual members as possible what he or she thinks are the three most important norms for the team? You should be sure he or she understands the term, *"norms."* In what way(s) are their responses similar to or different yours? Once you have tallied and analyzed the responses—share your findings with the team and discuss whether they feel the norms are helpful, or problematic and what might be needed to make the norms contribute to a more supportive team climate.

Video Discussion Exercise

Analyze the video

- *Apollo 13* (1995)

Interactive Simulation Exercise

Pagano, M. (2015). *Communication case studies for health care professionals: An applied approach* (2nd ed.). New York, NY: Springer Publishing Company.

- Chapter 9, "I've Got the License, So We're Doing It My Way" (pp. 91–100)

Health Care Issues in the Media

Health care as a team sport
https://www.ted.com/talks/eric_dishman_health_care_should_be_a_team_sport

Health Communication Outcomes

Interprofessional health care team communication is critical to 21st-century patient care and successful health organization goal attainment. Regardless of the type of health care facility, developing effective intra- and interprofessional teams is vital to accomplishing tasks, solving problems, and assuring collaborative decision making. In order to provide the best potential outcomes, several factors involving intra- and interprofessional health care teams need to be carefully addressed and analyzed, including team norms, roles, status differences, and relationships. Similarly, the importance of diversity to interprofessional health care teams, not merely in clinical roles, but with regard to sex, age, education, culture, and so forth. It is vital that health care teams use diversity to expand thinking, analysis, task completion, problem solving, and decision making. At the same time, these teams need to recognize that with diversity, including status differences and role distinctions, comes the potential for negative conflict. Consequently, interprofessional health care teams need to work to encourage positive conflict and maximize idea generation, input, and collaborative information sharing. In order to encourage this positive use of diversity and minimize the risk of groupthink, or negative conflict—health care teams should strive to create supportive team climates.

◾ REFERENCES

Benne, K., & Sheats, P. (1948). Functional roles of group members. *Journal of Social Issues, 4*, 41–49.

Tandy, C. (1992). Assessing the functions of supportive messages. *Communication Research, 19*, 175–192.

◾ BIBLIOGRAPHY

Campbell, S. H., Pagano, M., O'Shea, E. R., Connery, C., & Caron, C. (2013). The development of the Health Communication Assessment Tool: Enhancing relationships, empowerment and power-sharing skills. *Clinical Simulation in Nursing, 9*, e543–e550. Retrieved from http://dx.doi.org/10.1016/j.ecns.2013.04.016

Cragan, J., Kasch, C., & Wright, D. (2009). Communication in small groups: Theory, process, skills. In *Managing group conflict* (7th ed., pp. 243–275). Boston, MA: Wadsworth.

Engleberg, I., & Wynn, D. (2007). *Working in groups.* In *Verbal and nonverbal communication in groups* (4th ed., pp. 121–148). Boston, MA: Houghton Mifflin.

Hoover, J. (2005). Effective small group and team communication. In *Team decision making and problem solving: Types and procedures* (2nd ed., pp. 88–106). Belmont, CA: Thomson-Wadsworth.

Mannix, E., & Neale, M. (2005). What makes a difference? The promise and reality of diverse teams in organizations. *Psychological Science in the Public Interest, 6,* 31–55.

Rothwell, J. (2015). In mixed company: Communicating in small groups and teams. In *Roles in groups* (9th ed., pp. 134–162). Boston, MA: Cengage.

Weiss, D., Tilin, F., & Morgan, M. (2013). The interprofessional health care team: Leadership and development. In *Group development* (pp. 19–38). Sudbury, MA: Jones & Bartlett.

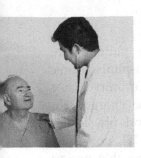

CHAPTER 10

Provider–Provider Communication

For the purpose of this text, we are going to use the following as working definitions:

- *Burnout:* Psychological and/or biological state in which employees feel stressed, overworked, and/or undervalued by the organization, other providers, and/or patients/families
- *Electronic health record (EHR):* Patient's Internet/cloud-/computer-based documentation of his or her past medical history, medications, allergies, and so forth
- *Electronic medical record (EMR):* Hospital, health care organization, and/or private provider's office documentation of patient's health care
- *Horizontal hierarchy:* Organizational communication that flows between members
- *Vertical hierarchy:* Organizational communication for those in leadership positions that generally flows downward to subordinates

■ HIERARCHY AND AUTONOMY

As discussed earlier, U.S. health care delivery has evolved over the past 100 years from a field of study that was almost totally dominated by physicians to a more corporate, team-focused culture. In the first 60 to 70 years of the 20th century, physicians worked in near absolute autonomy. They not only had solo or group practices, but they were the senior administrators in many of the nation's health care institutions. As a consequence, they were in a position to control much of what happened in health care from providers' roles, costs, treatments, hospitalizations, and regulations. Prior to the 1970s, there were various, generally local attempts to control health care delivery, but for the most part physicians were the decision makers—clinically, economically, and politically.

During these decades, physicians made nearly autonomous patient care decisions, including who needed which tests and treatments, hospitalizations, and so forth. This power and status offered physicians the opportunity to not just control patient care decision making and what would be charged for those services, but also command over physician–patient and physician–nonphysician (RN, physician assistant [PA], physical therapist [PT], etc.) communication. As a result, physician–provider interactions during this period were often as autocratic and paternalistic with nonphysician providers as they were with patients. Many MDs/DOs (doctors of osteopathy) perceived their advanced education and role as the basis for autonomous decision making and order giving in health care organizations. However, as discussed previously, with the rapidly increasing costs of health care delivery, political and economic factors were brought to bear in the name of managed care—to reduce insurance and government expenditures. Although managed care clearly limited physicians and midlevel providers' autonomy it also led to changes that both positively and negatively impacted health communication.

As physicians' and midlevel providers' (PAs and advanced practice registered nurses [APRNs]) decisions came under much more economic and clinical scrutiny with case managers and insurers' regulations, providers' communication behaviors became the lens that would be used to assess patient's care delivery and compensation. With the reductions in health care reimbursement for services, providers had to see more patients in order to meet either administrative policies, or their own financial needs. But just as provider–patient communication was impacted by managed care, so too was provider–provider.

Reflection 10.1. Think back to a recent health care visit, can you recall any provider behaviors that you think might have been related to managed care regulation? For example, did the provider seem rushed? Were you asked to come back on a different day for follow-up tests and/or treatments?

_____

_____

_____

_____

_____

With the increased scrutiny of all aspects of health care delivery, physicians and health care organizations had to reassess their policies, procedures, and communication approaches. Consequently, it became critically important, especially for hospitals, to identify ways to assure they would be financially solvent in spite of the insurance changes. For example, throughout much of the 20th century, it was not uncommon for a pregnant woman to have an uncomplicated delivery, vaginal or caesarean section (c-section), and remain in the hospital for 3 to 5 days even a week postpartum (after the birth). However, as insurers analyzed the data, they started to require that patients be sent home with in 2 days of an uncomplicated delivery. Therefore, hospitals that had been paid for 3 or more postpartum days were now losing thousands of dollars per patient. And any patients who stayed beyond the deadline determined by the insurer would be an additional loss for the institution for services provided that had to be collected from the patient—if allowed by the insurer, and/or economically feasible for the patient. In order to adapt, hospitals started requiring hospital-employed case managers and/or nursing staff to closely monitor patient stays, health documentation, and proposed treatments.

As one of the many results of managed care and increased insurance scrutiny of health care costs, provider–provider communication has evolved from a primarily vertical hierarchy (downward from physicians to nonphysicians), to a more horizontal hierarchy in which nonphysicians are much more participative and collaborative in patient treatment plans. As discussed in Chapter 9, team communication is the new norm in health care organizations. And although it could be argued that hospitals always used teams, the communication among team members, certainly in the first 75 years of the previous century, was overwhelmingly vertical from physicians, often conveyed in an autocratic style to nonphysician providers. Today, in order for everyone involved in patient care to be compensated, provider–provider communication has become not only necessary, but a requirement in many institutions. No longer can hospitals, for example, afford (financially) to have physicians admit patients without working closely with other providers to determine the most appropriate treatment plan, and how those decisions impact the insurer's authorized length of stay, reimbursement for services, and so on. Consequently, health care delivery economic realities have in large part forced changes in provider–provider team dynamics, but also in making communication more horizontal than vertical. Clearly, there is no disputing that physicians are legally responsible for the patient's diagnosis, treatment, and outcomes. However, no longer is that legal reality enough to provide physicians with decision-making autonomy. Patients today are demanding more information and increased input into their health care management. At the same time, hospitals and other organizations that employ physicians and/or grant nonemployed physicians privileges to admit patients and utilize the institution's resources, frequently—vis-à-vis their case managers—demand information and/or input into patients' treatment plans, especially regarding provider documentation and discharge timing. Therefore, although provider–provider communication in interprofessional patient care teams has moved toward a more horizontal hierarchy (except in life-or-death situations in which one person needs to take command) for patient assessment and treatment, other aspects of organizational provider–provider communication have in some ways spun 180° with nonphysician case managers making frequent demands of physicians regarding hospital-based services and discharge decisions. This evolving provider–provider hierarchy, both clinical and organizational, can be observed in face-to-face (F2F) interactions, but also in the electronic documentation of patient's hospital care.

■ ELECTRONIC MEDICAL RECORDS

As health care delivery has become more codified and regulated, provider–provider communication has evolved. Chapter 9 explored the changes in provider–provider team communication; however, it is important to understand how much of provider–provider information exchange is nonverbal. For much of the prior century, patient records were used to share patient information primarily between physicians and/or midlevel providers and to provide orders to be executed by nonphysicians. Although patient records have been required communication in U.S. hospitals since Franklin first documented that rule in 1754, only in the past 30 years have records taken on more extensive organizational and provider–provider information-sharing roles. Prior to the major shift in health care delivery in the 1980s providers shared information—intraprofessionally (doctor's notes, nurse's notes, etc.) via handwritten and/or dictated and transcribed paper records. Although there were clearly sections of the record that were interprofessional, "orders" were where prescribers (MD/DO, PA, APRN, certified registered nurse anesthetists [CRNAs], etc.) wrote instructions for nurses and others to fulfill. The records were considered legal documents intended to communicate patient information to other providers, primarily physicians, and orders. During this era, hospitals billed patients and eventually their insurers (or both) for the services provided—regardless of the patient's diagnosis. Consequently, if in 1965 a physician admitted a patient to the hospital with a diagnosis of pneumonia, the doctor could decide to do a barium enema (and either document the reason why or not) while the patient was hospitalized. Then, when the patient was discharged, the hospital would bill the insurance company for the patient's services, bed charge per day, lab tests, x-rays, and the barium enema and almost always the patient's insurance company would pay the bill—based on services provided. As you can see, the value of written patient records had a number of shortcomings:

1. Physicians frequently appeared to perceive the purpose of the record to be as a form of intrapersonal communication/information reminder for the author

2. Difficult to read/interpret because of penmanship/legibility issues related to physician handwriting

3. Lack of consistent and/or codified information documentation/sharing

4. More often, provider-focused, not patient-centered information

5. Primarily intraprofessional

Because the written medical record had so many problems for readers, it often, in order to be clearly understood, encouraged or required F2F or telephone provider–provider interactions; however, the realities for insurers were even more severe. Not only could payers frequently not decode the physician's handwriting or self-created abbreviations/symbols in order to understand the patient's complaint, history, signs, symptoms, exam findings, clinical assessment, and/or treatment plan—the insurers were either provided photocopies via the postal service, or facsimiles of medical records that frequently had their own technical issues causing even more reading/interpreting difficulties.

Reflection 10.2. Think about the process of writing. What is the difference for you in writing with a pen and paper versus typing? Which do you prefer and why? Which do you think enables you to communicate the same message faster?

_____

_____

_____

_____

_____

Consequently, it should not be surprising that for numerous reasons (first and foremost economic) the government required first hospitals and later provider offices to convert to EMRs if they wanted to continue to receive Medicare compensation. Faced with the potential loss of hundreds of millions of dollars over the long term, hospitals changed to EMRs (although, the electronic software was not developed to be used beyond the health care systems that purchased it).

As a result of the conversion to EMRs, health care institutions were able to quickly and easily search patient's records for billing to more clearly determine a patient's specific diagnosis, treatment, and/or plans as well as the detailed services provided by the institution. Early in the 1980s, diagnosis-related groups (DRGs) were developed to change the focus of hospital billing from a service perspective to a diagnosis approach. As such, providers needed to document a specific diagnosis and treatment plan so hospital/health care institutions could convert that to the appropriate DRG code. For example, a patient with abdominal pain had a much different DRG than a patient with a cholecystitis and cholecystectomy (inflamed gallbladder and gallbladder removal). And remember, the hospital will be paid not on the service, but on the diagnosis, so the more specific the DRG, the greater the likelihood the institution will receive a higher compensation. Consequently, provider–provider communication verbally and in EMRs is expected to clearly describe findings, interpretations, services provided, and treatment plans. And although there is still separate intraprofessional documentation in EMRs, these areas are used to assess patient care and to verify that all hospital costs are recorded and subsequently charged to the insurer and/or patient. As provider–provider communication evolved in EMR documentation, it has also created potential new problems in information sharing.

As part of hospital and The Joint Commission policies, providers are required to document their patient care in the EMR. And as has been discussed previously, the provider's record-keeping in an EMR can be problematic in terms of provider–patient communication, as well as patient perceptions of provider's focus and interest. However, provider–provider communication in EMRs has also suffered because of technology. One of the issues that many hospitals are dealing with is providers who use copy-and-paste features to circumvent their examination, communication, and assessment of the patient each time the patient is seen. And although it may seem like a good idea to copy and paste a complete history and physical from one day to the next, it does not aid provider–provider communication because readers cannot know what the provider observed, examined, and assessed longitudinally. Not unlike the problems with provider–provider communication in written records, which could not be read, or contained insufficient information, copied-and-pasted records—though legible—are of no value to readers who do not know what the current reality is versus prior documentation. It may be true that no change in a patient's condition seems to require very little provider–provider discussion in an EMR; however, the only way for another provider/reader to know what the basis is for the "no change" determination is for it to be supported by a reporting of exactly what occurred between the provider–author and the patient. The role of the EMR in horizontal provider–provider, as well as provider–hospital, and provider–insurer communication is critically important to the patient's care, but also to the institution's and the provider's reimbursement. As we have discussed here and in Chapter 9, EMR documentation and F2F provider–provider interactions are part of the health care system's communication approach intended to enhance intra- and interprofessional information sharing, analysis, decision making, and patient outcomes.

■ SYSTEMS APPROACHES

As discussed in Chapter 9, health care organizations, especially hospitals, rely on a systems approach to enhance interprofessional team communication. However, provider–provider information exchanges are also enhanced with a systems theory focus. When we think about intraprofessional health care teams, especially MD/DO and RN, but also laboratory, radiology, and other technicians, they need to work interdependently with professional peers to accomplish their patient care goals. For example, MD/DO intraprofessional provider–provider communication is needed for cross-discipline consultations (gastroenterologist-surgeon, cardiologist–pulmonologist, emergency medicine-infectious disease, etc.). Although the various board-certified specialists are experts within their disciplines, successful patient outcomes rely on intraprofessional provider–provider communication that is not obfuscated by miscommunication, roles, status, and so on. As previously mentioned, EMRs, if clearly and accurately authored to reflect what the provider knows, plans, and why—consultants will not have to rely on F2F provider–provider interactions as the major source of patient information. Similarly, status differences between intraprofessional providers have the potential to negatively impact the information shared by each interactant. Knowing that potential status differences could exist between a neurosurgeon and a pediatrician, for example, both professionals need to recognize this possibility and strive to communicate openly and completely without appearing elitist, subordinate, or superior. In order for both providers to share necessary data and analyses, each needs to work independently, but contribute interdependently. Just because one MD/DO provider has a different specialty than another—should only serve to enhance the interdependent outcomes of their collaboration.

Reflection 10.3. How does it make you feel when you are working for or with someone you feel has a higher status than you do? Not in terms of what you communicate, but how? Are you more concerned with how you say things? Do you think you are being judged because of the status differences? How do you think this would impact you if you were a health care provider working with another professional who you perceived to have a higher status?

_____

_____

_____

_____

Similarly, RNs need to communicate intraprofessionally (provider–provider) to assure that information is completely and clearly exchanged, but also that each interactant has an opportunity to provide/request feedback for clarification, understanding, and elimination of miscommunication. As mentioned previously, situation, background, assessment, and recommendation (SBAR) is a communication tool designed to help enhance provider–provider communication. However, effective use of SBAR and other provider–provider communication formats will only be as effective as the professionals who choose to use them. Consequently, providers need to understand the critically important nature of handoffs, from one RN to another, or to one hospitalist/resident/emergency department (ED) provider and so forth in order to assure that missing and/or miscommunication do not negatively impact patient care. Although after an 8- to 12-hour, or longer shift, it is clearly difficult to take extra time to ensure that patient information is clearly and effectively assimilated and understood. However, as discussed earlier, there is a difference between hearing something and understanding it correctly, so providers need to take the time to use feedback (both the sending professional and the receiving person) to clarify, enhance, and/or restate their messages.

As discussed in Chapter 9, a systems approach to health care interprofessional team communication relies on both effective intraprofessional provider–provider information sharing in order to positively contribute to interprofessional health care team interactions. Therefore, in order for interprofessional team members in the medical intensive care unit (MICU) to appropriately analyze a patient's infection, they must rely on the professional abilities of the microbiology technicians (MBT) to plate and maintain the patient's cultures, as well as analyze and correctly interpret the results. However, because it takes days for microbial cultures to grow and be tested, there is a high likelihood that more than one MBT will be involved. Therefore, effective intraprofessional, provider–provider communication will be necessary to ensure the accuracy of the data reported, as well as the positive impact of the intraprofessional lab team's contributions to the interprofessional patient care team's provider–provider communication. The interdependent nature of an organizational systems approach—with every member of the patient's health care team working independently but communicating and participating interdependently—provides the greatest opportunity for goal attainment and successful patient outcomes. However, although intra- and interprofessional provider–provider communication is critical to effective health care delivery. The various roles, status, norms, and realities of 21st-century patient care also frequently contribute to a higher level of professional burnout.

■ BURNOUT

As you may or may not know, stress and burnout are unfortunate realities for professionals working in U.S. health care delivery. And although there are numerous potential etiologies for these conditions, it is important that we explore how organizational and provider–provider communication may contribute to health care professionals' stress and/or burnout. As we have been discussing there are many demands and expectations for health care professionals regardless of their degrees, licenses, and roles. For example, hospitals must offer patient services 24/7/365; therefore, health care providers are frequently required to work diverse shifts of evenings, nights, and/or daytime schedules. And sometimes these shifts alternate during the same week. Consequently, not only can the change in sleep patterns for the providers involved (MD/DOs, RNs, PAs, APRNs, CRNAs, technicians, etc.) create stress, but the family of the health care provider is also impacted, such changes require adaptations by spouses/partners and/or children—not to mention day care, school issues, and so forth. But organizational schedules are far from the only stress inducers for health care professionals.

Among the many health communication, related causes of stress, beyond scheduling/sleep changes are:

- Power inequalities
- Status differences
- Clinical versus administrative conflicts
- Perceived peer pressure
- Emotional stress
- Ethical concerns

Reflection 10.4. Can you recall a stressful time in your life, how did that stress impact how you worked, studied, communicated? Why?

_____

_____

_____

_____

_____

For health care providers, there are both intra- and interprofessional stressors related to power and/or status issues. Whether it resonates from condescending, patronizing, or autocratic provider–provider communication, or from real or perceived status differences that discourage information sharing, questioning decisions, or providing diverse viewpoints—the results are often the same—increasingly stressed health care professionals who find it difficult to accomplish goals. For many providers, the stress of spending time on administrative, rather than clinical activities and communication can lead to professionals' self-doubt, frustration, and/or anxiety. Furthermore, some providers have described the stress they feel resulting from few if any communication outlets for discussing, intra- or interprofessionally, the emotional strain of caring for sick patients; their occasional feelings of inadequacy or ineptitude; a diminished sense of self-worth; and/or the sadness that accompanies the death (expected or not) of patients. But equally stress provoking can be the ethical issues that arise in provider–provider communication related to decision making, following orders, quality-of-life concerns, organizational versus clinical choices, and so forth. Clearly, effective provider–provider communication is critical to successful patient outcomes and organizational goal attainment.

However, provider–provider communication all too frequently ignores the individual needs of the human interactants and becomes as objective as the decisions they may be struggling to answer.

As we know, stress affects our thinking, morale, and often our communication effectiveness. But unfortunately, for far too many health care providers, the stress of 21st-century health care may lead to a sense of burnout and a decision to change careers/professions. Burnout is a serious problem for health care delivery and information sharing because it not only limits further the professional contributing to provider–provider communication—without the input from the departed person—but it also often increases the stress on the remaining health care professionals. Therefore, the remaining providers—with their own levels of stress—have to add to their workload and/or train a new team member to continue the expected excellent level of patient care in spite of the missing provider. However, although the loss of health care providers to other careers as a result of stress is a serious problem, it pales to the tragedy of suicide, which affects health care providers more than other professionals. Apparently, for some providers, the stress of modern U.S. health care delivery is too much and they choose suicide over communicating their issues to other providers, or changing careers. This tragic burnout reality is especially true for residents, MD/DOs, RNs, and other providers (see "Health Care Issues in the Media"). One of the goals of provider–provider communication should be to assess the interpersonal communication of the other interactant and use feedback and empathic listening to try to identify colleagues, intra- or interprofessionals, who are using communication behaviors (verbal and nonverbal) to demonstrate their stress, burnout, or suicidal ideations. Health care providers must recognize the risk of stress and burnout among patient caregivers (lay and professional) and seek to discover those who need help, whether they are patients, family members, or colleagues. Provider–provider communication is typically perceived as patient centered, but it also can be used to assess health care professional's emotional health as well.

Reflection 10.5. Have you been in a conversation with someone you knew and she or he was not behaving normally—was overly quiet, sad, or hostile? If so, what did you do? Did you inquire about the unusual nonverbal/verbal communication? If you haven't been in such a situation, how do you think you would respond to such an interaction? Why?

_____

_____

_____

_____

_____

Reflections (among the possible responses)

10.1. Think back to a recent health care visit, can you recall any provider behaviors that you think might have been related to managed care regulation? For example, did the provider seem rushed? Were you asked to come back on a different day for follow-up tests and/or treatments?

Very often, 21st-century health care delivery providers' communication behaviors can be observed and analyzed to see whether they appear to be influenced by issues external to the current provider–patient interaction. For example, because of the requirement to complete EMRs it is not uncommon for providers to have a *cow* in the exam room between himself or herself and the patient, or to be using a tablet or laptop similarly positioned. Consequently, the provider is often perceived by patients to be paying more attention to the computer nonverbally, than to the patient. In addition, because of the provider's time demands, to see a certain number of patients per day, or in a prescribed time limit, may use behaviors that communicate to patients that the provider is in a hurry, for example, interrupting the patient or changing the subject. In some cases, providers may be examining patients while seeking information, even asking questions while auscultating a patient's chest or abdomen. Similarly, patients frequently complain of the provider's asking for feedback while clearly in the process of closing the conversation. These nonverbal and verbal behaviors may relate to the provider's disease-focused approach, but in all likelihood they are in some way related to meeting the provider's economic and managed care goals. Because of reduced reimbursement for patient visits by Medicare and private health insurers, providers need to see more patients each day to maintain their billable visits.

10.2. Think about the process of writing. What is the difference for you in writing with a pen and paper versus typing? Which do you prefer and why? Which do you think enables you to communicate the same message faster?

For many writers, there is a distinct difference between using a pen and paper and a computer/tablet for creating documents (medical and nonmedical). Some authors like the feel of writing, others like the keyboard. However, for providers, the advantages of the EMR are numerous: it is easy to use, allows space-less storage versus paper records, and it is legible, archivable, and consistent. However, the problems for provider authors center on the use of a computer in the provider–patient interaction and the noise and distraction it causes in the communication channel. Furthermore, the lack of a standardized interhospital format, let alone nationally, contributes to the provider–provider communication difficulties with use of diverse formats, checklists, and so forth. Consequently, without a single format throughout U.S. health care, providers are still forced to print out a patient's records and fax them to another provider, or risk privacy issues if they try to e-mail a patient's EMR to a consulting or new provider.

10.3. How does it make you feel when you are working for or with someone who you feel has a higher status than you do? Not in terms of what you communicate, but how? Are you more concerned with how you say things? Do you think you are being judged because of the status differences? How do you think this would impact you if you were a health care provider working with another professional who you perceived to have a higher status?

In general, when Americans are communicating with someone who is perceived to have a higher status, the lower status interactant communicates less, defers more, and is less likely to raise new issues. In provider– provider communication, these realities can create serious problems for patient care, information sharing, analysis, collaboration, and decision making. Unfortunately, for many providers status differences in health care still persist, MD:RN, MD:PA, MD:APRN, RN:technician, and so forth. It can be hypothesized that these perceived distinctions are education/ certification/license based; however, many providers use status to take a more authoritarian/paternalistic approach to provider–provider communication. Consequently, health care professionals in intra- and/or interprofessional communication contexts must strive to minimize status differences through their verbal and nonverbal behaviors (encouraging discussions and diverse viewpoints/ideas; not interrupting; using proxemics and kinesics to show interest; not dominance, power, or control). Although status differences may be real, they can be minimized in provider–provider communication if both interactants work to enhance the information sharing and goal attainment vis-à-vis collaborative and participative discourse in a supportive climate.

10.4. Can you recall a stressful time in your life? How did that stress impact how you worked, studied, communicated? Why?

If you are like most of us—stress impacts all aspects of our lives. Many people feel stress has both biological and emotional repercussions. For example, stress has been shown to contribute to headaches, stomach issues (gastroesophageal reflux disease [GERD], peptic ulcer disease [PUD], etc.), malaise (tiredness), and even immune system disturbances. In addition, stress can cause emotional changes such as difficulty concentrating, lack of interest or heightened emotional responses (anger, sadness, etc.). Consequently, when a health care professional feels stress, he or she may withdraw from participating or reduce his or her involvement in provider–provider and team communication. Therefore, stressed providers may limit their professional role by calling in sick more frequently than usual or refusing to work extra shifts, staying later, and so on. Stress could negatively impact a health care provider's intra- and interprofessional provider–provider and/or team communication.

10.5. Have you been in a conversation with someone you knew was not behaving normally—was overly quiet, or sad, or hostile? If so, what did you do? Did you inquire about the unusual nonverbal/verbal communication? If you haven't been in such a situation, how do you think you would respond to such an interaction? Why?

It can be very disconcerting to be in a conversation with someone you know who is not communicating as he or she normally would. Frequently, friends or lovers will ask the other person, "What's wrong? You don't seem like yourself!" Sometimes these queries will get a response that indicates the person understands the situation and expects it to change. Or the person will elaborate on the cause of the unusual behavior. Either of these responses can be helpful in encouraging a person, especially a health provider colleague, understand the reasons for the behavioral change. And that understanding can be used to assess whether there is reason for concern regarding an overstressed provider who needs some professional help. However, sometimes stressed-out individuals are so upset that they cannot or will not communicate what they are feeling and why they are behaving differently than usual.

Regardless of the provider's response, you should consider communicating your observations to the other person and encourage him or her to talk about the problem/issue with you, or to a qualified professional. Clearly, if you have concerns that a colleague may be severely stressed and his or her communication behaviors lead you to believe that he or she may have suicidal ideations, you should seek out qualified help. Generally, provider–provider communication is intended to enhance a patient's diagnosis, treatment, and outcomes, but it should be remembered that providers are no different than nonproviders in terms of needing health care themselves from time to time. Provider–provider interactions are a good opportunity to assess other provider's stress levels and, if necessary, to assist him or her in finding help. The suicide rates among health care professionals highlight the potential for provider–provider communication to help identify and aid those with significant stress/emotional problems.

Skills Exercise

Go to a professor you know, or a supervisor at work, and ask him or her how he or she handles peer–peer/professional–professional communication with someone who has a higher status (perceived or stated) in the organization. Ask the person what criteria he or she uses to assess the status of a colleague beyond a title or role. Also, try to determine whether the individual has any examples of perceived status differences with someone who had a similar organizational title and why he or she felt the distinctions existed. How would this person recommend overcoming them to enhance peer–peer organizational communication and goal attainment? What are some of the recommendations that might be helpful to a health care professional in a provider–provider interaction with someone of a different status?

Video Discussion Exercise

Analyze the video

- *The Hospital* (1981)

Interactive Simulation Exercise

Pagano, M. (2015). *Communication case studies for health care professionals: An applied approach* (2nd ed.). New York, NY: Springer Publishing Company.

- Chapter 2, "See One, Do One, Teach One" (pp. 17–26)
- Chapter 9, "I've Got the License, So We're Doing It My Way" (pp. 91–100)
- Chapter 32, "You'll Feel Better Recovering at Home" (pp. 309–318)

Health Care Issues in the Media

Stress, burnout, and suicide
http://www.nytimes.com/2014/09/05/opinion/why-do-doctors-commit-suicide.html?smid=nytcore-ipad-share&smprod=nytcore-ipad&_r=1

Health Communication Outcomes

Provider–provider intra- and interprofessional communication, either dyadic or in health care teams, is critical to successful 21st-century health care and provider and organizational goal attainment. In most U.S. hospitals and other health care institutions, provider–provider interactions follow a systems theory approach in which communicators work independently (professionally, clinically, and/or administratively) to accomplish their roles, tasks, and goals, but are expected to share information, analyses, and so forth interdependently to maximize the opportunities to provide the most effective, safe, and economically appropriate patient care possible. One of the major channels for provider–provider communication is EMR information sharing.

With federal mandates for hospitals and other health care organizations to convert from ink and paper to EMRs—provider–provider communication has been significantly impacted. First, EMRs assure legibility for provider (and other) readers of patient records. Second, intraorganizationally, EMRs offer providers near-instant access to patients' health information. Third, EMRs can be readily updated with patient reports from tests, procedures, and consultations (labs, x-rays, surgeries, etc.) for providers (intra- and interprofessional) to utilize in their patient care analysis and decision making. However, with electronic record keeping there are also provider–provider as well as provider–organization communication issues.

1. Patient privacy: Access possible by any organizational provider
2. Information sharing: EMRs are not standardized, so one hospital's requirements for documentation of provider communication may be very

different from another. For example, one institution may focus nearly entirely on checklist responses with few expectations or requirements for narratives versus another hospital's EMR, which uses more narrative than checklist responses.

3. Quality of provider posts: Within the same organization, providers are generally free to determine what information to document. Too often, providers choose to copy and paste prior documentation from 1 day to the next. Therefore, with a string of similar, if not exact provider notes—it is nearly impossible for another provider to know what the realities of the provider–author's examination and analysis of the patient's condition are.

4. Logistics: One of the major flaws with EMRs currently is they are not universally accessible. Consequently, what a provider documents in the EMR in his or her office or hospital cannot be electronically viewed by a provider not associated with that private office and/or hospital.

Therefore, provider–provider communication via EMRs can be very beneficial, frustrating, or inaccessible. However, provider–provider discourse can also be negatively impacted in F2F conversations based on status differences between the interactants (intra- or interprofessionally).

One of the major roadblocks to effective provider–provider communication is related to perceived or real status differences between the health care professionals (intra- or more often interprofessional). Status differences clearly can negatively impact interpersonal discourse; however, in provider–provider dyadic or health care team communication for interprofessionals there are at the very least education, certification, and/or licensure differences—MD/DO and RNs; APRNs and RNs, MD/DO and PAs/APRNs, MDs/RNs/APRNs/PA and physical therapists/laboratory and/or radiology technicians, and so forth. Of course there are potential status differences intraprofessionally as well based on clinical specialty, honors/awards/publications, and/or administrative titles (chief of medicine, chief of nursing, chair of neurosurgery department, etc.). A key problem with status differences in provider–provider interactions is that the person who feels of less status frequently is less communicative, shares less information, provides less feedback, tends to use a groupthink approach, and may be unwilling to offer new ideas or diverse thinking. Consequently, it is important for providers (intra- and interprofessionally) to recognize the risks associated with perceived or real status differences in interpersonal and team health communication in order to minimize or eliminate the negative consequences of such verbal and nonverbal behaviors on patient care. All of these aspects of provider–provider communication are critical to effective health care delivery; however, in addition to the potential benefits such information exchanges have for patients and organizations—provider–provider communication also offers an opportunity to identify and address a provider's stress and burnout as well as more life-threatening emotional issues.

Provider–provider communication can also be used to assess the impact of stress and/or burnout on health care providers and address it before it becomes a serious personal and/or organizational issue—especially when a provider may see drug/alcohol abuse or suicide as the only solution to his or her stressful situation. There is an axiom in communication, humans cannot, *not* communicate! Consequently, verbally and nonverbally we are always communicating. Therefore, your artifacts—clothes, hair, jewelry, body art, and so forth—are communicating about you to others. So too when people who are usually outgoing and communicative suddenly become withdrawn and less responsive, they are communicating those realities whether they intend to or not, but only if other interactants are listening/looking. Therefore, more providers can use their clinical lens not only to observe patients' verbal and nonverbal behaviors, but also colleagues' communication cues to assess whether there are signs that more information needs to be gleaned about the provider's stress, feelings, actions, and ideations. Provider–provider communication, although generally less frequently examined, is a critically important aspect of successful health care delivery, organizational goal attainment, as well as safe and effective patient care.

■ REFERENCE

Franklin, B. (1754). *Some account of the Pennsylvania hospital: From its first rise to the beginning.* Philadelphia, PA: Franklin & Hall.

■ BIBLIOGRAPHY

Kongstvedt, P. (2013). *Essentials of managed health care* (6th ed.). Burlington, MA: Jones & Bartlett.

Kreps, G. (1990). Applied health communication research. In D. O'Hair & G. Kreps (Eds.), *Applied communication theory and research* (pp. 313–330). Hillsdale, NJ: Lawrence Erlbaum.

Orbe, M., & King, G. (2000). Negotiating the tension between policy and reality: Exploring nurses' communication about organizational wrongdoing. *Health Communication, 12*(1), 41–61.

Pagano, M. (2011). *Authoring patient records: An interactive guide.* Sudbury, MA: Jones & Bartlett.

Thomas, E., Sexton, J., & Helmreich, R. (2003). Discrepant attitudes about teamwork among critical care nurses and physicians. *Critical Care Medicine, 31*(3), 956–959.

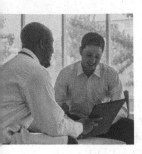

CHAPTER 11

Health Care Leadership Communication

For the purpose of this text, we are going to use the following as working definitions:

- *Contingency theory:* A leader is determined by the situation and how well his or her style/skills match the current needs—identifying which behaviors are best suited for a variety of contingencies

- *Leader–member exchange (LMX) theory:* Leaders are not making decisions in order to impact followers, they are trying to collaborate with followers; the communication between a leader and his or her followers

- *Leadership:* The ability of one person to persuade a team and/or organization to accomplish agreed-upon goals

- *Path–goal theory:* A theory based on how leaders persuade followers to accomplish goals

- *Situational approach:* Leaders adapt their approaches based on the situation, including their employees' skills and knowledge

- *Skills approach:* A management style that is leader focused, not personality driven, but talents and skills can be learned

- *Styles approach:* A management style that is leader focused, not personality driven, and highlights leaders' behaviors and how their communication impacts followers based on the context

- *Team leadership:* Leaders working within teams to accomplish goals

- *Trait approach:* A management style that is leader-centric and emphasizes that certain people are born with explicit personality traits that make them leaders; with this approach, leaders are born, not made

■ TRAITS, SKILLS, AND STYLES

Health care leadership in the 21st century has evolved in countless ways. In America, for most of the country's history, patients and other providers viewed physicians as the leaders in health care delivery. Whether it was in their private offices, at the hospital bedside, or in health care administrative roles— physicians were perceived as the central figures in patient care. And although physicians continue to be critically important to the current interprofessional health care team system—U.S. health care takes much more of a group—than an individual-centric approach. Consequently, U.S. health care moves to more collaborative communication goals (patients, intra- and interprofessional teams, organizations) in order to improve patients' outcomes. Therefore, the examples in prior decades of physicians' and other providers' autocratic, paternalistic leadership communication (with patients, providers, and administrators) needs to be supplanted by a more collaborative, supportive, and engaging style in provider–provider, provider–patient, and provider–organization communication.

Early in the 20th-century, leadership was thought to be primarily based on inborn traits. Leaders were believed to have unique personality qualities and characteristics that separated them from others and were the reason for their leadership roles. However, as more research was done, it became obvious that leadership was not some type of genetic predisposition that limited who could be a potential visionary/manager, but instead was based on a wide variety of factors that could be learned (socially, academically, and/or professionally). As you can imagine, if indeed leaders had to born with the skills, knowledge, and abilities needed to persuade followers and create new opportunities—this chapter would be unnecessary and very few Americans would be considered leaders. However, the trait approach has identified some key traits or characteristics that may be important for successful leaders, including:

- Knowledge
- Self-assurance
- Persistence
- Honesty
- Amiability

Although these traits are important for leaders to possess in varying degrees, it is obvious that most of these are personal values that are developed or intelligence that includes both education and experience—but not things humans are uniquely born with. As you know from your own lives— leadership occurs in diverse ways. It is important to understand that leaders can be assigned (appointed or elected) as in the chief of surgery, or the surgical intensive care unit nurse manager, and so forth. Or they can emerge, based on their behaviors, skills, and communication, to assume a leadership role. For example, there could be an interprofessional team assigned to create the content for a hospital's new electronic medical record (EMR). And although there may, or may not be, a leader appointed to direct this team, it would not be uncommon for a member of the team, through his or her efforts, intellect, and communication, to emerge as the person the team actually views as its leader and seeks direction and feedback from.

The question for health care providers who will be working in teams—but also at various times with patients, families, and peers as leaders—is how do effective leaders communicate and persuade followers to accomplish shared goals? As you may have surmised from the title of this chapter—the key to accomplishing leadership goals as well as team and organization goals is always effective communication. Regardless of the tasks, problems, needs, or goals, if more than one person is working to accomplish them—persuasive/collaborative interpersonal and team communication are going to be critical. Therefore, potential health care provider leaders need to understand the differences and benefits of various communication skills and styles.

Although there are a variety of theories related to the most beneficial leadership skills, it seems clear that they all share several key components, including:

1. Personality/humanism
2. Knowledge/judgment
3. Vision/communication

One of the skills that have been identified as important for effective leaders is the ability to work well with others and participate with them in accomplishing goals. This humanist aspect of leadership is important to developing interpersonal relationships and trust with members/followers, but needs to also be supported by the person's knowledge (education and experience) as well as his or her ability to analyze information and make necessary decisions. However, depending on the role, context, and goals, a leader may need to have a vision for others to follow, but regardless, the leader's success and effectiveness will depend on his or her leadership and interpersonal communication skills. But, in addition to the role traits and skills play in leadership, the communication styles a leader adapts will also be important to his or her success.

Reflection 11.1. Consider someone in your life you consider an effective and/or successful leader (parent, professor, professional) and try to identify what specifically (traits, styles, and/or skills) about his or her behaviors contributed to his or her leadership. Why?

_____

_____

_____

_____

_____

Although traits and skills are predominantly about a leader's personality, values, knowledge, visions, and social abilities—leadership style is focused more on communication behaviors. For example, as discussed earlier in this chapter and others, the use of a paternalistic/authoritarian communication approach to health communication is one of the styles leaders can use to try to persuade followers/patients/peers/other providers. Consequently, a leader who uses a paternalistic style is focusing on giving orders and therefore the result becomes the major emphasis for both leader and follower(s). An opposite style is much more focused on followers and their needs, but the task/goal becomes secondary. One of the most collaborative styles for health care providers to consider is a team management approach that focuses on interdependence, with relationship building, goal attainment, and shared respect between leader and followers. However, there are other leadership communication theories for health care providers to understand and potentially apply in their various roles, situations, and/or teams.

■ CONTINGENCY, PATH–GOAL, AND LMX THEORIES

As health care professionals who are likely leaders in many different contexts (family, intraprofessional, interprofessional, etc.), it is important to not just recognize that individual characteristics are important to effective leadership; interpersonal, cultural, and organizational theories are also useful. For example, you likely know someone who possesses many of the traits, styles, and skills that have been identified as important for leadership—and yet the individual was not as successful as expected.

Contingency Theory

At its most basic, contingency theory is about identifying the most appropriate leader for a specific context. In health care, for example, contingency theory suggests that there are certain situations in which just because a person has a specific title, degree, and/or license—he or she may not be the ideal person to be the leader. This can be seen in 21st-century health care administration, where many of the senior administrators/leaders in hospitals and other health care systems are not physicians, nurses, and so forth. As the context for health care organizational

Reflection 11.2. Can you see the distinction between contingency theory and situational theory? Try to recall an example for each, whether in your life, in history, or the media, and discuss how it applies to these different theoretical approaches to leadership.

_____

_____

_____

_____

_____

leadership has evolved from primarily a clinical context to a more business-model approach—leadership has changed as well.

It is important to recognize that using a contingency-theory approach, leaders would be appointed or chosen based on their abilities to either focus on a goal(s) versus interpersonal relationship development. Therefore, by recognizing a leader's strength in task completion or interpersonal development, based on the situation—the most effective leader can be determined. Consequently, where previously any leader with certain traits, skills, and styles was felt to be a potential leader in any context, contingency theory points out that to be most successful it is very important to match a leader's strengths to a situation's needs/demands. Therefore, a leader is not expected to be universally the ideal choice for every context. Thus, a non-provider chief executive officer (CEO) of a health care system may be the best leader administratively, but clearly not the best leader in a clinical crisis (e.g., mass casualties from a motor vehicle accident [MVA]) in the hospital's emergency department (ED). The importance of contingency theory for health care professionals is that it should remind you that based on the context a leader may need to be selected, appointed, or emerge who has the most appropriate task or relational traits, skills, and styles to address the situation—regardless of his or her title, degree, and so forth. Although this book will not go into detail about the differences between contingency and situational theories, the major distinctions are that in situational leadership, the leader seeks to align his or her approach to the followers' abilities based on the context. For example, a chief nursing officer (CNO) might choose to be more authoritarian in a situation that included many newly graduated RNs, versus another contex in which more experienced RNs were dealing with a similar problem but need more collaboration and support, rather than instructions or orders. As you can see, contingency theory is primarily focused on the leader's skills/styles as they relate directly to the circumstances. Whereas the situational approach links the leader's choices not just to the context, but to his or her followers' abilities and commitments. Just as these two theories provide differing perspectives for health care providers to use in determining the best leadership approach to follow so too does path–goal theory.

Path–Goal Theory

As the name implies, a path–goal approach to leadership relies on a leader identifying the most appropriate style to use to persuade his or her followers to attain a shared goal. Path–goal theory focuses on a leader helping subordinates understand the organization's/team's goal, helping followers determine the best path to attaining it, using his or her role to minimize or eliminate any obstructions, and collaborating with the team as needed for a successful outcome. The role of motivator is key for leaders who utilize a path–goal approach to problem solving/goal attainment, and so forth. Some of the specific behaviors needed by leaders for path–goal theory, based on their followers' needs and the task/goal include:

- Giving orders or specific instructions
- Providing support and encouragement
- Collaborating/participating

Consequently, in a hospital, for example, a leader using path–goal theory might need to be more autocratic in communicating with members exactly how to reach a goal of 100% for the unit's handwashing—"Be sure to wash your hands before you enter every patient's room and when you leave; there will be monitors watching you." Or, with a different group, the leader might choose to be more encouraging and supportive—"I know you can help us reach our 100% handwashing goal because you are committed to patient safety and our success." Finally, the leader might decide to collaborate with a team based on their characteristics to help identify a way to reach the goal—"I would like to work with you all to develop a plan that will help us assure we reach our 100% handwashing goal; together we can make it a reality."

As you can see from these examples, in path–goal theory leaders are not just focused on the outcome, but on analyzing their followers/subordinates to determine the best leadership styles and skills to use to motivate them to succeed. This move toward leadership that addresses not just organizational problems, tasks, and goals, but analysis of the subordinates as well, contributes to another important leadership concept—LMX theory.

LMX Theory

Compared to the theories described earlier, LMX theory is focused on the communication between a leader and his or her followers/subordinates. One of the key elements in LMX theory is the understanding of motivated teams versus nonmotivated groups. By identifying those subordinates

Reflection 11.3. Have you ever worked in a group or on a team where some members would do anything to help achieve the shared goals, but others were not as motivated? If so, who did you identify with in the group/team—those who were motivated or not motivated? Why? How did your choice impact the group/team's outcome, as well as your perceptions of working with that group/team? If you have not been in such a situation, how would you hypothesize it might impact a leader's communication behaviors to have motivated and unmotivated subordinates?.

who are motivated and willing to do what is needed regardless of role/job descriptions, leaders can develop more effective interpersonal communication and relationships with those who are motivated to help them attain goals, complete tasks, and solve problems.

As you may have surmised, one of the realities of LMX theory is that those who are in motivated groups not only get more interactions with organizational leaders, but also tend to be identified and promoted to become future leaders. Consequently, LMX theory provides a way not just for current leaders to behave, but a plan to help prospective leaders demonstrate their interest, commitment, and contributions to the organization, its leaders, and its goals. Suppose you were a hospital unit manager and of the 20 employees under your leadership, five are always willing to accept new tasks, help solve problems, or fill in when other members are unavailable. Who are you more likely to want to work with when you have a problem or a new goal to accomplish, the five motivated members, or those who are not? Similarly, when asked by your supervisor who you would recommend for a promotion to a leadership position, does it not make perfect sense based on an LMX approach that the recommendation will come from the motivated group, even if that person might have less seniority than a member of the unmotivated group? Therefore, LMX theory helps leaders identify followers who may be best equipped to help problem solve, complete tasks, and attain goals based on their motivation, but also be the best choice for future leadership roles within the organization. However, in addition to LMX, path–goal, situational, and contingency theories—it is critically important for health care providers and professionals to understand the differences and benefits associated with team leadership theory.

Team Leadership Theory

As we have discussed throughout this text, U.S. health care delivery is predominantly based on a team approach—even within a private practice setting there is often an intraoffice team as well as various interoffice teams (e.g., consultants, service providers, even institutions). Consequently, one of the most important leadership theories for health care professionals is team leadership. However, team leadership does not exist in a vacuum—therefore, a team leader needs to understand the previously discussed theories, traits, skills, and styles and utilize them appropriately based on the context, team members, and goals. In addition, effective team leaders need to be continually monitoring both the context they are functioning in as well as the team's progress toward an intended outcome/goal. Some of the specific activities that team leaders need to focus on include:

- Assuring goal understanding
- Strategizing for success
- Encouraging shared decision making
- Providing information and/or materials to help the team accomplish a task/goal

- Communicating interpersonally with members
- Managing conflict
- Exemplifying the commitment, ethical behavior, and excellence that is expected from members

As these actions illustrate, team communication is both dyadic and group focused. Team leaders need to develop interpersonal relationships with their members, but also be able to communicate effectively with all members in order to assure there is not a feeling of favoritism or bias. As discussed in Chapter 9, team communication is critical to 21st-century U.S. health care and how team leaders choose to use their interactions with the group and individual members will determine in large part how the team performs and whether tasks/goals are effectively accomplished and patient care enhanced. Clearly, because the purpose for most health care teams, whether intra- or interprofessional, are task, problem solving, and/or goal related—a team leader needs to carefully assess the situation, his or her team members, and the outcome that is needed. However, as important to health care as team leadership and team communication are, understanding the role of women and leadership in health organizations is also vital.

Women and Leadership

Although it may seem odd to single out women and leadership, there are a number of reasons why this is important to understand:

1. More women than ever before are working in U.S. health care today.

2. Increasingly, there are greater numbers of female versus male providers (MD/DO, RN, advanced practice registered nurse [APRN], physician assistant [PA], etc.) graduating every year from U.S. health professions programs.

3. Important distinctions in leadership behaviors are based on sex and gender.

4. Almost always, more women are working as health care providers in U.S. health care delivery institutions than are males.

5. Inaccurate misperceptions exist regarding the stereotype of an American female leader.

It has been shown that women leaders tend to be more collaborative than males; however, there does not appear to be any significant difference in the sexes when it comes to interpersonal and task-related styles. And the two sexes seem equally effective in leadership roles. Therefore, with increasing numbers of female health care providers in all professions/disciplines, it is important for peers to understand the realities about women in health care leadership and ignore inaccurate stereotypes.

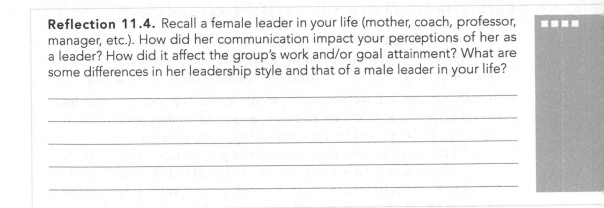

Reflection 11.4. Recall a female leader in your life (mother, coach, professor, manager, etc.). How did her communication impact your perceptions of her as a leader? How did it affect the group's work and/or goal attainment? What are some differences in her leadership style and that of a male leader in your life?

Female health care provider leaders need to be assessed like their male counterparts, on their results and ability to motivate followers and attain organizational goals. Although it is a sad truism in 21st-century America, that even though women are earning more academic degrees than males, they continue to be paid less for the same job as their male counterparts. For example, according to Cain Miller (2016) in the *New York Times*, "Women who are surgeons earn 71% of what men earn" (para. 3). However, this disparity between modern health care professionals based on sex is not limited to salaries. According to Torrieri (2014), "women account for 73% of medical and health services managers, but only account for 18% of US hospital CEOs" (para. 1). This inequity is hard to believe; however, for U.S. female health providers it is no less a reality.

From a leadership communication perspective, female health care professionals must understand the current situation and recognize how increasing leadership by women can only serve to enhance the opportunities for others. Similarly, although female providers might analyze the data presented earlier and hypothesize that using masculine-gendered behaviors (aggression, independence, competitiveness, etc.) would be the path of least resistance to higher leadership positions—a reassessment of interpersonal relationships, health, and leadership communication realities would be very helpful. For example, feminine-gendered individuals, regardless of sex, are generally more collaborative, participative, and nurturing. These feminine-gendered skills/styles are exactly what have been recommended in numerous leadership theories. Consequently, rather than trying to be like male leaders in their communication behaviors, health provider females who seek leadership roles need to focus on mentors whom they view as most effective, regardless of the leader's sex. And they need to recognize the importance of choosing the right leadership approach based on the context, members, goals, and tasks. With more women successful in leadership roles across all different types of organizations, will the barriers to female leadership begin to dissolve and stereotypes be forgotten? Women health care providers are in the majority and, with continued effort and effective interpersonal, organizational, team, and leadership communication, they will assume the leadership roles they deserve.

11.1. Consider someone in your life you consider an effective and/or successful leader (parent, professor, professional) and try to identify what specifically (traits, styles, and/or skills) about his or her behaviors contributed to his or her leadership. Why?

Generally, you may have been able to recognize the role that the leader's knowledge, personality, communication, and collaborative style played in his or her success. Often, we identify someone as an effective leader if we feel that we have a relationship with that person—not just as one of many working on a project, but someone he or she knows and cares about on some level. We are more open to persuasion and efforts to reach goals if we feel valued and that everyone is sharing in the work, but also when we are recognized for our contributions. Finally, most Americans prefer collaborative, rather than authoritative leadership styles—we want to be part of something, not just ordered to do things. And this participative approach leads to a sense of individual and team ownership of the shared tasks, problem solving, and goal.

11.2. Can you see the distinction between contingency theory and situational theory? Try to recall an example for each, whether in your life, in history, or the media, and discuss how it applies to these different theoretical approaches to leadership.

One historical example would be General George S. Patton. In World War II, General Patton was known as a very authoritarian leader. He used a very masculine-gendered, independent, aggressive, and competitive approach to persuading/commanding his troops. When General Dwight D. Eisenhower appointed General Patton to his leadership post we can hypothesize that it was in part related to contingency theory—the U.S. tank battalions were getting beaten by the Germans—a leader with charisma and confidence was needed to take charge of the situation. Only a few years later, when the war was over and the context was different, General Patton was removed from his post for being too independent and aggressive in his comments to the press. Consequently, we can see how contingency theory helps us understand how different contexts call for different leaders and/or leadership skills and styles.

11.3. Have you ever worked in a group or on a team where some members would do anything to help achieve the shared goals, but others were not as motivated? If so, who did you identify with in the group/team—those who were motivated or not motivated, and why? How did your choice impact the group/team's outcome, as well as your perceptions of working with that group/team? If you have not been in such a situation, how would you hypothesize it might impact a leader's communication behaviors to have motivated and unmotivated subordinates?

Based on the situation, members' motivations play a major role in leadership behaviors. As LMX theory suggests, when some members choose to do just the bare minimum of work and seem less invested in the task, problem-solving effort, and/or goal—it is likely they will not be perceived as motivated employees/teammates and consequently the organizational leader will pay less attention to them and more to those who are enthusiastic and committed. Consequently, the motivated members will be given more opportunities for input into the decision-making and goal-attainment efforts, as well as frequently identified as ideal leadership candidates when organizational opportunities arise.

11.4. Recall a female leader in your life (mother, coach, professor, manager, etc.). How did her communication impact your perceptions of her as a leader? How did it affect the group's work and/or goal attainment? What are some differences in her leadership style and that of a male leader in your life?

Female leaders, like males, can choose to communicate using either masculine- or feminine-gendered behaviors. And regardless of their sex they would be wise to decide which communication approach is needed based on the context, members, and goal. However, because female leaders have been shown to be more collaborative and participative in their leadership styles, it would not be surprising if that is what you observed in many of your experiences. Often, leaders who are not directive, but participative in their communication with members, are perceived as being more interpersonal and relational in their style and may verbally or nonverbally encourage others to behave similarly. Among the differences in leadership that you might have observed were more listening and nurturing communication behaviors by feminine-gendered leaders, as well as the aforementioned efforts to collaborate and participate in tasks, problem solving, goal attainment, and so forth. As with the trait approach that focused on leaders being born with the needed leadership characteristics, skills, and styles, it is important to avoid the U.S. stereotypical view of males being more appropriate in leadership roles than females. Again, there is no evidence to support that genetic differences between the sexes make one more suitable for leadership than the other. Avoid stereotypes in both your views of what makes a successful and effective leader and your openness to leadership, regardless of the individual's sex or gender. Instead of stereotyping, use his or her behaviors, ethics, and outcomes to inform your analysis.

Skills Exercise

In an organization (family, academic, or professional) or team in which you are an active member, analyze a current or recent task and/or goal that your teammates/family were assigned to successfully accomplish. Focus your analysis on the leader's (yours if you were the leader) communication behaviors and how he or she tried to persuade members to complete the task/goal. What leadership theory, styles, traits, and skills did you see as being most beneficial (from leader and follower perspectives)? How did the context for the group/team effort impact leadership and followers behavior? In what ways did the sex and/or gender (of both the leader and followers) affect the effort and outcome? From this analysis, how will you consider your own health care leadership choices?

Video Discussion Exercise

Analyze the video

- *Patch Adams* (1998)

Interactive Simulation Exercise

Pagano, M. (2015). *Communication case studies for health care professionals: An applied approach* (2nd ed.). New York, NY: Springer Publishing Company.

- Chapter 9, "I've Got the License, So We're Doing It My Way" (pp. 91–100)

Health Care Issues in the Media

The costs of health care
https://www.youtube.com/watch?v=iEXkKV3kbb8

Women as hospital CEOs
http://www.healthcaredive.com/news/why-women-account-for-just-a-fraction-of-hospital-ceos/337822

Health Communication Outcomes

Leadership communication is critical to the success of 21st-century providers, teams, and organizations. However, to be effective and successful health care leaders and professionals need to understand that certain personality traits are important to possess, but a leader does not have to be born with them. Traits, like leadership skills and styles, can be learned from family, peers, mentors, academics, and life experiences. However, based on the theoretical approach to leadership chosen, a leader may need to utilize a variety of traits, skills, and styles depending on the context, task, problem, goal, and his or her followers/members.

Contingency theory, for example, requires leaders to be chosen or appointed based on the task, problem to be solved, and/or goal. Therefore, it is goal driven, with the choice of leader relating to his or her expertise, skills, styles, and education most appropriate for the context. In contrast, situational theory is more follower focused in that the leader tries to align his or her style with the members' abilities in order to address the situational goal. In contrast, path–goal theory is leader focused and suggests that to attain a goal the leader needs to identify the most effective way to motivate his or her members/followers, remove obstacles, and support their efforts. Using a different focus, LMX theory seeks to use the followers' motivations as the lens for a leader to use in determining which members to focus his or her communication toward. Therefore, a leader who uses LMX theory, in order to accomplish tasks, solve problems, generate ideas, and attain goals, seeks to identify the most motivated members of the organization or team and work primarily with them to complete the assignment/goal. In addition, LMX theory provides an opportunity for an organization/team to identify potential future leaders based on their level of motivation and efforts.

Although each of these theories has potential for health care provider leaders, team leadership may be the most commonly used form in day-to-day health care delivery. Because so much of 21st-century health care is done in team environments, intra- and interprofessionally, leadership in health care organizations generally falls into two distinct, but interdependent macroteams: administrative and clinical. However, team leadership theory is applicable to both and generally includes one of the other theoretical perspectives based on the leader, members, tasks, and so forth. Based on team leadership theory, a leader needs to be very communication-centric (interpersonal and team) and analyze both the goal and his or her teammates to provide understanding, motivation, and feedback, but also to offer support, conflict management, ethical behaviors and a collaborative, participative environment for the maximum sharing of information, ideas, and solutions. Finally, especially in modern health care organizations, it is important to note the increasing roles and numbers of women in all health professions and the need to concomitantly expand their leadership roles—both clinically and administratively. Consequently, stereotypes of female professionals need to be avoided and gendered communication behaviors, regardless of a person's sex, need to be analyzed to determine the ideal leader for the task, problem, situation, team, and goal. By understanding the various leadership theories discussed in this chapter you should be able to identify not only the best choice for you as a future leader, but also understand that leadership is not dependent on a person's genes (inherited traits and/or sex), but on how an individual uses his or her education and life experiences to develop the necessary personality characteristics, skills, and styles of a successful and effective leader.

■ REFERENCES

Cain Miller, C. (2016, January 15). How to bridge that stubborn pay gap. *New York Times*. Retrieved from http://www.nytimes.com/2016/01/17/upshot/how-to-bridge-that-stubborn-pay-gap.html?_r=0

Torrieri, M. (2014). *Why women account for just a fraction of hospital CEOs*. Retrieved from http://www.healthcaredive.com/news/why-women -account-for-just-a-fraction-of-hospital-ceos/337822

■ BIBLIOGRAPHY

Aronson, E. (2001). Integrating leadership styles and ethical perspectives. *Canadian Journal of Administrative Sciences, 18*(4), 244–256.

Avolio, B., & Locke, E. (2002). Contrasting different philosophies of leader motivation: Altruism versus egoism. *Leadership Quarterly, 13*, 169–191.

Graeff, C. (1997). Evolution of situational leadership theory: A critical review. *Leadership Quarterly, 8*(2), 153–170.

Lee, A. (2010). Who are the opinion leaders? The physicians, pharmacists, patients, and direct-to-consumer prescription drug advertising. *Journal of Health Communication, 15*, 629–655.

Northouse, P. (2013). *Leadership: Theory and practice* (6th ed.). Thousand Oaks, CA: Sage.

Wageman, R., Fisher, C., & Hackman, J. (2009). Leading teams when the time is right: Finding the best moments to act. *Organizational Dynamics, 38*(3), 192–203.

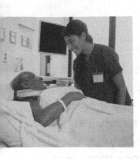

CHAPTER 12

Risk Management and Health Communication

Canera L. Pagano

For the purpose of this text, we are going to use the following as working definitions:

- *Adverse event:* Injury or harm to a patient that is the result of medical care and treatment and may or may not have been preventable

- *Disclosure:* A process of informing patients and family members about the occurrence of an adverse event

- *Incident reporting:* A system or process in which staff members identify events that are out of the norm for routine care of patients or hospital operations, for example, a patient or visitor who falls in the hospital

- *Never event:* A term used to identify certain adverse events that are preventable and not reimbursed through Medicare

- *Risk management:* A method of identifying, assessing, and reducing risk and/or harm to patients, visitors, and staff as well as reducing the risk of financial loss to the organization

■ CHANGING THE LANDSCAPE OF RISK MANAGEMENT

Risk management in the health care setting can trace its origins from other industries, such as manufacturing, where the focus of the risk manager was on transferring risk through the purchase of insurance. With his or her knowledge of the insurance industry, the risk manager's responsibilities included purchasing insurance, ensuring that adequate coverage was maintained to cover loss, and reporting claims to the insurance carrier for handling and resolution. In addition to claims reporting, risk managers also have a claims management role once a patient sustains injury or a lawsuit has been filed against the organization or provider. Typically, these activities revolved around investigating events after they occurred and developing strategies to defend the organization in the event of a lawsuit. Once the lawsuit was filed, the risk manager would retain outside counsel to handle the matter and assist in identifying witnesses and gathering documents or other evidence to be used in defense of the organization. With their knowledge of claims, risk managers were able to identify certain high-risk areas and tasks on which they could focus preventative activities in an effort to avoid lawsuits and the resulting financial and reputational losses to the organization.

Reflection 12.1. Think about your home; what are some of the risks to visitors, service providers (postal employee, contractors, etc.), and/or the building/property that you as a renter or owner must be aware of and try to minimize and/or cover with homeowner's or renter's insurance? How might those risks be increased in health care organizations?

_____

_____

_____

_____

_____

The 1998 Institute of Medicine (IOM) report *To Err Is Human* made public what risk managers and health care providers have known for decades—patients suffer preventable harm in our health care institutions. The report further demonstrated that these errors come with not only a high financial cost but also a significant cost in terms of patient harm. With the publication of the report came greater demands for transparency, including public reporting requirements for infections resulting from ventilator use, central lines, and urinary catheters. In addition, many states publicly report the number of adverse events that occur in hospitals, such as falls, medication errors, and surgical events, including wrong-site surgeries or retained foreign bodies (surgical instruments, sponges, etc.). In addition, data related to patient surveys are also publicly reported. Therefore, if they are aware, the public can use this information to compare different medical institutions and individual providers based on how well they communicate with patients, respond to concerns, and manage certain health conditions.

Because of the IOM report and changing health care costs, risk managers are becoming more and more involved in patient safety initiatives. Many of these enterprises focus on errors as a result of system failures as opposed to focusing on individual clinical decision making or the failure to follow policies and/or procedures. The focus on system failures has prompted many health care institutions to adopt behaviors and processes that are associated with highly reliable non–health care organizations. These behaviors and processes have been taken from industries, such as aviation and the nuclear power industry, and adapted by hospitals to improve their patient safety and provider–patient, provider–provider, and provider–organization communication. The use of situation, background, assessment, and resolution (SBAR) and three-way repeat back (e.g., I give you information, you repeat it back to me, and I confirm that you have correctly assimilated and communicated it) are meant to improve provider–provider information exchanges as well as offer a mechanism for ensuring patient safety through the use of code words (e.g., "I have a concern" or "let me clarify") that alert a provider to a potential safety issue/miscommunication.

Changes in health care and in how health care providers communicate through electronic media have been beneficial in terms of availability and access to information; however, they have also brought challenges for risk managers. The advent of electronic medical records, the almost universal availability of smartphones, and social media have created areas of risk that were previously unheard of in the health care setting. As health care continues to evolve, the focus of the risk manager increasingly expands to include these new technologies and their potential impact on patient safety and promoting health care organizational transparency while protecting the institution against loss. Clearly, for risk managers, the need to problem solve by gathering information, analyzing it, conferring with appropriate organizational members to assess risk and developing, sharing, and reassessing policies/procedures to minimize it—are all dependent on institutional members' effective interpersonal, team, and organizational communication. However, in addition to the individual organization's risk-management communication, information must also be shared with regulatory bodies.

■ ADVERSE EVENTS: STATE AND FEDERAL OVERSIGHT

There is very little doubt that health care is one of the most heavily regulated industries in existence. The intersections of state and federal agencies that regulate and monitor modern health care are numerous. Furthermore, each agency has its own standards or rules and reporting mechanisms by which health care providers and organizations must abide and communicate compliance. Failure to comply (organization or provider) can result in monetary fines, loss of licensure, and possibly incarceration.

Because of such broad oversight, it is not uncommon for a health care organization's adverse event to potentially trigger reviews by multiple agencies. Typically, the state, through a public health role, has oversight for safety and care provided to patients in hospitals. In their public safety role, the state utilizes different statutes, codes, and regulations to set forth requirements for hospital organization, staffing, and patient safety. In addition, the state mandates reporting of certain events such as child abuse and neglect, gunshot wounds, and the reporting of communicable diseases. Furthermore, a growing number of states mandate the reporting of certain adverse events.

A 2008 review by the Office of Inspector General (OIG) revealed that over half of all states had mandated adverse event reporting. Of those states, nearly half utilized the National Quality Forum (NQF) List of Serious Reportable Events or some variation of the list as the basis for reporting. The NQF has identified nearly 30 incidents that fall into the following event categories:

- Surgical
- Product or device
- Patient protection
- Care management
- Environmental
- Criminal

The occurrence of any one of these events needs to be appropriately communicated and can result in a cascade of regulatory investigations, findings, and potential violations.

For example, a hospital that finds itself in the position of having to report a wrong-site surgery, medication error that results in death, or a fracture from a fall may be faced with an investigation by the state public health agency. The state has the authority to issue violations or fines, and restrict or revoke a health care organization's licensure. In addition to investigating the institution, the state may use the occurrence of an adverse event as the impetuous to investigate an individual provider and possibly take action against him or her by issuing a fine and restricting or revoking the provider's professional license. Furthermore, the same adverse event that triggered a state investigation may trigger an investigation under federal regulations by a federal agency.

Hospitals that are reimbursed for treating patients covered by Medicare must comply with the Conditions of Participation (COP) established by the Centers for Medicare & Medicaid Services (CMS). These regulations and conditions provide the framework and parameters for how hospitals deliver care to patients. Consequently, a wrong-site surgery will not only trigger an investigation by the state but may also trigger an investigation by CMS under the COP. A violation of the COP can result in a monetary fine or, depending on the seriousness of the event, the hospital could be placed in immediate jeopardy of being terminated from the Medicare program unless an immediate corrective action is put in place. For most hospitals, termination from the Medicare program would be financially disastrous.

Furthermore, an adverse event that results in a state and federal investigation could also result in an inquiry by The Joint Commission (TJC). TJC accredits approximately 21,000 health care organizations. Accreditation by TJC is a seal of approval for health care organizations for Medicare certification. The deeming authority of TJC allows hospitals to be certified to deliver care to Medicare recipients without having to undergo a separate federal survey. Not surprising, accreditation under TJC can be in jeopardy as a result of a "sentinel" or adverse event. TJC defines a *sentinel event* as a patient safety occurrence that results in death, permanent harm, or severe temporary harm such that intervention is needed to preserve life. TJC defines these events as sentinel events because the occurrence of such an event signifies the need for an immediate investigation and corrective action. It is important to highlight that adverse event reporting is a required organizational communication function and how the organization communicates the problem, its analysis of the situation, how it developed and implemented the corrective plan, as well as follow-up steps to assure the plan is successful or needs further revision will determine TJC, state, and/or federal responses. Although it may seem obvious, it is vital to note that generally, adverse events result from miscommunication, absent communication, or communication that is not followed (policies and procedures); however, the only way to effectively address the regulatory investigations and corrective action plans related to a sentinel event is through successful provider–provider and provider–organization communication. It is well established that risks can result from verbal and/or nonverbal provider–provider or provider–patient communication behaviors. But in 21st-century health care delivery, when risks become adverse events providers and organizations are being encouraged to communicate what happened to the affected patient and/or family.

> **Reflection 12.2.** When you think about adverse events, incorrect medication, wrong-site surgery, slip and falls, and so forth, how do you see provider–patient and/or provider–provider communication being critical to reducing these risks and/or developing policies/procedures to minimize or eliminate their occurrences?
>
> _____
>
> _____
>
> _____
>
> _____
>
> _____

■ DISCLOSURE OF ADVERSE EVENTS

The role of communication in the management of adverse events is truly a 360° review process that comes full circle when it is time to disclose to a patient or family that an unintended/unexpected event has occurred. These sensitive conversations require careful analysis, effective communication, and planning in order to be successful. Several states and large health care systems (see Brigham and Women's Hospital link in the "Health Care Issues in the Media" section) have developed their own disclosure processes and programs. Regardless of the source, these plans have numerous common features to promote disclosure of adverse events and to guide providers' verbal and nonverbal communication content when having these difficult conversations.

One of the first elements of a disclosure plan is to communicate the belief that ethically speaking, disclosure is the right thing to do. The American Medical Association (AMA) ethics opinion clearly states that patients have the right to be informed of their past and current medical condition and events that impact current and future care. This right is without regard to the physician's fear of liability or the filing of a lawsuit. It is the ethical obligation of the provider to communicate in an open and honest fashion with the patient and to explain in understandable terms the actions that resulted in the adverse event or unexpected outcome.

The other common feature among disclosure programs is the understanding that disclosure conversations require interdisciplinary investigation and preparation. Disclosure is not a single conversation but is instead a process in which multiple conversations, generally with diverse health professionals, are used to assess what occurred, why, and how to clearly communicate that understanding to the patient and/or family. Many disclosure programs recommend the use of a disclosure coach to help role-play the disclosure conversation and ensure that the communication to the patient is timely and conveyed with empathy, compassion and in understandable terms.

Disclosure conversations should take place very soon after an adverse event has been identified. Ideally within 24 hours of discovery of the unexpected/ unintended incident. Waiting to disclose until all of the facts are known is discouraged. It is critical to thoroughly investigate the event. However, the fact that an investigation is ongoing should not be a deterrent to disclosure. It is appropriate to disclose initial facts with a promise to return for further discussion as the investigation continues.

Providers need to remember that information disclosed to the patient should include a factual statement of what happened in patient-appropriate language. The provider should avoid stating that he or she is guessing or making assumptions about the cause of an event as this only leads to confusion on the part of the patient and family. In addition, if you make an assumption about how or why an event happened and the investigation reveals something different, the patient will not be confident that the real cause of the event was discovered or disclosed.

Another common feature of disclosure programs is recognition that not all adverse events are the result of practitioner or system error. As a result it is important to make a distinction between statements of sympathy versus an apology. If, after the investigation is completed and it is determined that the care and treatment of the patient was within the standard of care, then at the time of disclosure a statement of sympathy is appropriate. If, however, it is determined that the adverse event was the result of medical error, then a sincere apology should be offered. Once the apology is made there needs to be a plan for ongoing care of the patient and a plan for continued communication between the parties needs to be established. The patient needs to know whom he or she can contact regarding continuing care, concerns about billing, and compensation. It is important to understand that it is strongly advised that these conversations include thoughtful planning and consultation with risk management and other organizational professionals before making a statement of sympathy or apology.

> **Reflection 12.3.** What if you were a patient and you were given the wrong medication and became seriously ill? What would you want the health care provider/organization to communicate to you? How can the provider and the organization regain your trust and confidence? Why?
>
> _____
>
> _____
>
> _____
>
> _____

Finally, successful disclosure programs recognize that not only does the patient need support during an adverse event, but the health care providers who were involved in the incident also need support as well. Many disclosure programs include support processes to help providers—as they are too often forgotten victims—who may be dealing with feelings of guilt and shame after an adverse event. Although disclosure can be a helpful form of communication for providers as well as patients, disruptive provider communication can only create more stress and problems for colleagues, organizations, and/or patients.

■ COMMUNICATION PROBLEMS: WHEN BEHAVIOR BECOMES A RISK

Like other workplace environments, health care organizations have their share of employment issues. Claims of discrimination based on race, religion, gender, age, sexual orientation, and disability are not uncommon. Given the emphasis on patient safety and heavy regulatory oversight, health care organizations are particularly susceptible to claims of retaliation and whistle-blowing. Of particular concern are disruptive, verbal, nonverbal, and/or hostile behaviors by physicians, nurses, and other members of the health care team and their impact on provider–provider communication and patient safety. In addition, disruptive behavior creates a hostile work environment that perpetuates the cycle of troublesome conduct.

According to TJC, communication failures have been identified as one of the most frequently cited root causes in the sentinel events reported to the agency. It is not surprising that communication failures between health care providers result in patient harm. As a consequence, there has been a significant amount of nationwide emphasis placed on improving communication among members of the health care team. Some of these verbal and nonverbal recommendations include:

1. Identifying look-alike and sound-alike medications
2. Use of phonetic and numeric communication tools
3. Structured handoffs for transitions of care
4. Utilization of a time out in the operating room to prevent wrong-site/wrong-patient surgeries

However, despite concentrated efforts to improve provider–provider communication in the health care setting, communication errors continue to occur. One reason for communication failures is disruptive behavior.

Disruptive behavior is any conduct/communication that undermines the culture of safety in an organization. Specifically, behaviors that show disrespect or demean other members of the health care team and/or undermine the culture of safety that so many hospitals strive to create. Disruptive behavior includes a range of actions from the overt—such as yelling, the use of profanity, and throwing instruments or other items—to behaviors that are more passive–aggressive such refusing to speak to or acknowledge a particular member of the team. Although physicians are more frequently identified as engaging in disruptive behavior, other providers, such as nurses and pharmacists, have also been known to engage in problematic conduct. As you might hypothesize, the cause of disruptive behavior is not always clear. It may be the result of stress in the workplace or at home. It could also be the related to the pressure of working in a fast-paced often high-stakes (life or death) environment. Although the cause may not always be clear, the impact of disruptive behavior on teamwork and collaboration is unmistakably demonstrated in the way it impairs provider–provider and/or provider–organization, if not provider–patient communication.

Reflection 12.4. Recall a time when you were around a friend, coworker, supervisor, professor, or teammate who used disruptive behavior to either dominate the situation or to attack others to illustrate his or her power. How did the person's conduct impact the team/group/organization? How did you feel about participating in events with that person and why?

_____

_____

_____

_____

_____

Staff members who feel threatened, disrespected, and/or demeaned are more likely to make an error when providing patient care. Disruptive behavior also distracts the attention of well-intended staff members from a patient/ task focus to the problem provider. Such a scenario requires impacted providers to not only monitor a patient, they are also placed in the position of having to monitor the disruptive health care professional by being on alert for any telltale signs of an imminent outburst or nonverbal reaction. Therefore, disruptive behavior reinforces the hierarchical nature of medicine. Staff members who have been subjected to disruptive behavior tend to exhibit increased communication apprehension and are therefore less likely to speak up when they have concerns about patient safety because of a climate (team and/or organizational) of intimidation and fear created by the disruptive provider.

It is interesting to note that the different communication styles between physicians and nurses have been identified as a contributing factor in incidents of disruptive behavior. Physicians and nurses receive very different training in terms of communication. Physicians are trained to be problem solvers and to present information in an organized succinct manner so the problem and plan for a solution are easily identified. Nurses, on the other hand, are trained to be historians of the patient record. They are expected to assimilate a breadth of patient-related information and document it in minute detail in order to capture every aspect of a patient's care. These differences in roles and communication styles between providers can lead to stress, frustration, and/or burnout for the various professionals. Physicians may be frustrated because the nurse provides too much detail and information that is perceived to be irrelevant to physician decision making. The nurse could become frustrated because he or she perceives the physician as not listening or caring about the information being communicated. Therefore, a health care provider in either of these situations might communicate inappropriately and use a nonverbal or verbal disruptive behavior.

In order to bridge the differing communication styles, information-sharing tools have been developed that are intended to meet the needs of diverse health care professionals. One tool that is commonly used is the SBAR format. The use of SBAR allows nurses to provide pertinent historical information that is relevant to the issue to be resolved. For the physician, SBAR provides a brief concise description of the problem to be solved followed with either a recommendation or request for change in therapy or action to be taken. Although found to be beneficial to enhancing provider–provider communication, not all behavioral problems can be solved through the use of an information-sharing tool. When disruptive conduct continues, hospitals frequently resort to enforcing codes of conduct or the utilization of chain-of-command policies in order to escalate and address continued disruptive behavior. As a consequence, the onus is on health care providers to recognize the inappropriateness of disruptive behaviors in hospitals or other patient organizations and to utilize their interpersonal and team communication to enhance, not detract from their provider–provider interpersonal relationships and patient care goals.

Reflections (among the possible responses)

12.1. Think about your home; what are some of the risks to visitors, service providers (postal employee, contractors, etc.), and/or the building/property that you as a renter or owner must be aware of and try to minimize and/or cover with homeowner's or renter's insurance? How might those risks be increased in health care organizations?

Homes have a number of obvious risks for visitors. For example, a slippery sidewalk or a spilled beverage on the stairs. Even a tree that might be damaged and fall on a neighbor or in his or her yard. It is the homeowner's responsibility to minimize and/or eliminate these risks and also obtain insurance in case a risk turns into an injured visitor. Similarly, health care organizations must assess their institutional risks and not only purchase insurance to cover such events, if they occur, but do all they can to minimize or eliminate them. That is the major job of a risk manager.

12.2. When you think about adverse events, incorrect medication, wrong-site surgery, slip and falls, and so forth, how do you see provider–patient and/or provider–provider communication being critical to reducing these risks and/or developing policies/procedures to minimize or eliminate their occurrences?

Just as communication is almost certainly at the core of the adverse event—miscommunication, missing communication, and/or fictitious information—effective interdisciplinary health/team/organizational communication is required to identify the problem, analyze its cause, and develop a solution as well as a plan to reevaluate the process/procedure once it has been changed. The critical role of risk management is not only recognizing the problem, but in putting together an interdisciplinary team to effectively analyze it and develop a solution, which is all based on effective provider–provider and provider–organization communication. Although it is unthinkable that a patient might have the wrong leg amputated, it would be far worse if every effort was not made to understand how it happened and analyze the best approach possible to minimize the possibility that it ever happens again. Therefore, the important role of risk management in 21st-century health care centers not on just preventing risks through effective provider–provider and provider–organization communication, but in developing solutions to prevent recurrences. Through the use of appropriately selected interprofessional health care providers and administrators, an adverse event can be carefully analyzed and a solution clearly communicated vis-à-vis a process/policy/procedure that minimizes or eliminates similar potential risks.

12.3. What if you were a patient and you were given the wrong medication and became seriously ill? What would you want the health care provider/organization to communicate to you? How can the provider and the organization regain your trust and confidence? Why?

In all likelihood, if you were given the wrong medication and suffered an adverse event, your first responses, once you got better, would be confusion, anger, and distrust of the provider who administered it, but perhaps of the hospital as well. And in all likelihood you would want to know what happened. How it happened? And why it happened? A decade or more ago, it would have been fairly routine in a hospital not to answer any of those questions. In part, this reluctance to share information with a harmed patient was felt to be necessary to protect the provider and/or hospital from increased legal risk. However, current thinking supports the ethical obligation of a provider/ organization to inform the patient and/or family with as much information as is known about what happened, how, and why. In addition, from a provider– patient interpersonal relationship perspective—trust will likely not be possible if the patient feels information is being hidden. Trust relies on accurate and clear communication—especially in a situation in which a person has been harmed by the actions of another or an organization.

12.4. Recall a time when you were around a friend, coworker, supervisor, professor, or teammate who used disruptive behavior to either dominate the situation or to attack others to illustrate his or her power. How did the person's conduct impact the team/ group/organization? How did you feel about participating in events with that person and why?

Unfortunately, in health care organizations disruptive communication occurs all too often. Whether it is nonverbal behaviors like throwing things, making loud noises, or inappropriate gestures and/or responses—or verbal aggression in which one provider insults another, uses derogatory or inflammatory language, or sexist, racial, or ethnic slurs—inappropriate conduct by health care professionals is counterproductive to dyadic, team, and organizational goals and interpersonal relationships. Perhaps in response to this reflection you recalled a time when a professor or another individual in a position of power used verbal and/or nonverbal behaviors to disrupt the setting, as well as the goals of those in it. Generally, when such a scenario ensues, regardless of the organization—the conduct of the perpetrator is perceived by participants as both inappropriate and undermining the roles and goals of the team/ organization. In fact, it is not uncommon for disruptive behavior to enhance that person's sense of control—as others in the team/organization choose to communicate less with the disruptive individual.

Skills Exercise

You are a health care provider (MD/DO [doctor of osteopathy], physician assistant [PA], advanced practice registered nurse [APRN], RN, or pharmacist) working in a hospital and one of your patients, Jennifer Jones, has suffered from an adverse event—she was given the wrong medication, had a severe reaction, and is in the intensive care unit. Based on this reality, what risk-management/communication steps (be as specific as possible) would be needed in this situation? And, if it turns out the adverse event was caused by a miscommunication related to your order (MD/DO, APRN, PA), administration (MD/DO, APRN, PA, RN), or fulfillment (pharmacist)—how would you prepare to disclose that to Ms. Jones (if she's healthy enough) and/or her family?

Video Discussion Exercise

Analyze the video

- *House M.D.* "Nobody's Fault" (2012)

Interactive Simulation Exercise

Pagano, M. (2015). *Communication case studies for health care professionals: An applied approach* (2nd ed.). New York, NY: Springer Publishing Company.

- Chapter 29, "You Posted What on Facebook?" (pp. 283–292)
- Chapter 38, "Health Insurance Portability and Accountability Act (HIPAA)" (pp. 367–374)

Health Care Issues in the Media

Doctor–nurse behavior
https://www.ache.org/policy/doctornursebehavior.pdf

Adverse event disclosure
http://www.brighamandwomens.org/medical_professionals/career/cpps/ApologyDisclosure.aspx

Health Communication Outcomes

Risk management, though first started in other professions, has become a critically important aspect of health care delivery for organizations, providers, and patients. The goals for risk management are to use effective communication—verbal, nonverbal, and written—to minimize and, where possible, eliminate risks for patients, as well as for providers and, health care organizations. However, in order to lower risks, risk managers and organizational members (providers and administrators) must work together to identify potential risks, as well as develop a cause analysis for incidents and/or adverse events when they occur—and a corrective action plan, policies, and procedures to use to prevent/minimize any future recurrences.

In order to accomplish a health care organization's risk-management goalsgoals, effective interpersonal, team, and organizational communications are critical. Every member of a hospital, for example, needs to be aware of the policies and procedures in place to reduce risks, but also to understand the reporting requirements and steps if an incident or adverse event occurs. Adverse events can be extremely detrimental to patients (wrong-site surgery, medication errors, etc.), but also to the organization and its providers. Because health care incidents and adverse events are so often a function of provider–provider and/or provider–patient, communication, a number of critical tools and policies have been developed to try to improve the accurate transfer of information from one provider to another. For example, SBAR is used in many hospitals to enhance intra- and interprofessional provider–provider communication during a patient handoff and/or transfer, from one unit to another (e.g., RN–RN) and/or from provider to provider at shift changes (e.g., PA–APRN, or MD–PR/APRN). In addition, using a three-way repeat-back (360° feedback) process to better ensure a message was assimilated and interpreted correctly offers another provider–provider communication approach to enhancing not just the transfer of information, but the assessment of the other provider's understanding of the sender's message. However, in spite of risk-management policies, procedures, training materials, and communicationcommunication tools, adverse events still occur far too frequently in American health care organizations and when they do impacted patients and their families need to be informed.

The disclosure of adverse events to affected patients and/or their families has become an important part of risk management in American hospitals. Although informing those seriously impacted by unexpected or unintended consequences of care is the ethically responsible thing to do, it is also a wise behavior from a health communication/interpersonal relationship perspective. Providers need patients and their families to trust their abilities, information, and collaborative decision making. Therefore, although it is never easy to tell someone that an adverse event has occurred and what is known about its impact on the patient's health, it is necessary from ethical, as well as interpersonal communication/research foci. Perhaps, with disclosure and relationship building, trust can be restored between the provider–patient. And although disclosure communication needs to be carefully analyzed and discussed with the risk manager and other clinical and administrative members of a hospital/health care organization, it is important to understand that only what is known, not speculation, should be communicated—as soon after the event as possible. When more information is uncovered by cause analysis and other efforts, those details can be communicated at a later time. However, in the immediate post-adverse event period, the patient and his or her family need to be given information about who to contact with questions related to costs of care and next steps. But, in addition to reducing risk in health care organizations through policies, procedures, risk-cause analysis, and disclosure, risk managers also seek to eliminate provider–provider and/or organizationally disruptive communication (verbal and/or nonverbal) behaviors.

Because of perceived power and/or role differences, stress, and burn-out health care providers can resort to inappropriate interpersonal/team/organizational communication. This disruptive conduct can take the form of verbal attacks against one person or a team, or nonverbally through a variety of antisocial behaviors targeted at one or members of a health care organization. For example, there have been reported instances of surgeons throwing instruments either at a member of the surgical team or around the operating room. Similarly, some providers have been documented shouting profanities at colleagues, or being verbally aggressive toward organizational members (providers or administrators). As you can imagine, these disruptive behaviors create additional health care risks as members seek to avoid interacting with the disruptive provider and/or refuse to share information with him or her in an effort to reduce the risk of a tirade or other unprofessional conduct. Therefore, as patient care can be negatively impacted by providers' disruptive behaviordisruptive behaviors, the risk of an incident or adverse event increases for an organization. As a consequence, it is important for all members of an organization not to use disruptive communication, and, if aware of it, report it to a supervisor, risk manager, or human resources as soon as possible. This chapter has discussed health care risks and their management vis-à-vis effective verbal, nonverbal, and written communication policies, procedures, cause analysis, disclosure, and the elimination of disruptive provider behaviors. However, only through the interdependent, interprofessional, interpersonal/team/organizational communication and actions of all health care providers and administrators can patient/provider/organizational risks be reduced and/or eliminated.

■ BIBLIOGRAPHY

American College of Obstetricians and Gynecologists. (2012). *Committee opinion. Number 520: Disclosure and discussion of adverse events.* Retrieved from http://www.acog.org/-/media/Committee-Opinions/Committee-on-Patient-Safety-and-Quality-Improvement/co520.pdf?dmc=1&ts=20141202T0103275418

American Medical Association. (1994). *Opinion 8.12–Patient information.* Retrieved from http://www.ama-assn.org/ama/pub/physician-resources/medical-ethics/code-medical-ethics/opinion812.page?

Beckett, C. D, & Kipnis, G. (2009). Collaborative communication: Integrating SBAR to improve quality/patient safety outcomes. *Journal for Healthcare Quality, 31*(5), 19–28.

Department of Health & Human Services, Office of Inspector General. (2008). *Adverse events in hospitals: State reporting system.* Retrieved from http://oig.hhs.gov/oei/reports/oei-06-07-00471.pdf

Institute for Safe Medication Practices. (2012). *Raising the index of suspicion: Red flags that represent credible threats to patient safety.* Retrieved from https://www.ismp.org/newsletters/acutecare/showarticle.aspx?id=27

Institute for Safe Medication Practices. (2014). *Part II: Disrespectful behaviors: Their impact, why they arise and persist and how to address them.* Retrieved from http://www.ismp.org/Newsletters/acutecare/showarticle.aspx?id=78

Kavaler, F., & Alexander, R. (2014). *Risk management in healthcare institutions: Limiting liability and enhancing care* (3rd ed.). Burlington, MA: Jones & Bartlett.

Kohn, L., Corrigan, J., & Donaldson, M. (Eds.). (2000). *To err is human: Building a safer health system*. Washington, DC: National Academies Press.

Ristuccia, H., & Epps, D. (2009). Becoming risk intelligent. *Risk Management, 56,* 88.

Rosenstein, A., & O'Daniel, M. (2009). *How to identify and manage problem behaviors*. Retrieved from https://psnet.ahrq.gov/perspectives/perspective/82/how-to-identify-and-manage-problem-behaviors

The Joint Commission. (2016). *Hospital accreditation*. Retrieved from http://www.jointcommission.org/accreditation/hospitals.aspx

Wagner, S., & Layton, M. (2007). The two faces of risk: Cultivating risk intelligence for competitive advantage. *Deloitte Review, 1,* 71–75.

Youngberg, B. (2011). *Principles of risk management and patient safety*. Sudbury, MA: Jones & Bartlett.

Youngberg, B. (2013). *Patient safety handbook* (2nd ed.). Burlington, MA: Jones & Bartlett.

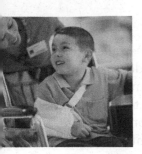

CHAPTER 13

Medical Malpractice and Health Communication

Canera L. Pagano

For the purpose of this text, we are going to use the following as working definitions:

- *Adverse event:* Injury or harm to a patient that is the result of medical care and treatment that may or may not have been preventable

- *Evidence:* Facts or material items used to support one side or another's theory of a case in a lawsuit

- *Harm:* Unexpected injury/illness resulting from negligence/an adverse event in treatment/care

- *Malpractice:* Negligence on the part of a professional

- *Negligence:* Failure to act as a reasonably prudent person would in the same or similar situation

- *Root-cause analysis:* Process of interprofessional analysis (usually intraorganizational) of an adverse event to determine the ultimate/root cause and contributing factors that resulted in harm to a patient(s)

■ COMMUNICATION IN MEDICAL MALPRACTICE

Because malpractice in health care is related to provider–patient and/or organizational patient communication/procedures/services, patients can suffer harm as a result of negligence in many different ways. Communication—whether it is provider–patient, provider–provider, or organizational—is frequently at the heart of the case. Research has indicated that the root cause of medical error in nearly two thirds of all malpractice claims was the result of ineffective communication. As a result, it is not uncommon to see allegations in a complaint for medical malpractice that focus on provider–patient or provider–provider communication. These allegations focus mainly on the failure of the provider to communicate important information to the patient, or ineffective provider–provider patient-related information exchanges. Although there are many examples of misinformation, no information, or unclear messages communicated to patients, allegations concerning communication failures between members of the health care team can also form the basis of a medical malpractice action. As a result, it is important for health care providers to not only focus on effective interpersonal and health communication exchanges with patients, but they must also remember that it is just as critical to practice those same communication skills when sharing information intra- and interprofessionally. As discussed in prior chapters, the need for multifocal approaches to effective provider communication should underscore the importance of provider–patient relationship building and how it can impact a patient's perceptions of not just his or her provider, but of how she or he will respond if an adverse event occurs.

Patients report dissatisfaction with the physician–patient relationship when they feel that their concerns are not being heard and/or taken seriously. Patients who perceive that their provider is misleading them in some way or not fully informing them of possible consequences of treatment are more likely to seek legal advice when treatment outcomes/prognoses do not go well or as planned. In addition, when providers fail to disclose adverse events to patients the patient is often left with the perception that the provider is attempting to hide something in addition to not being honest and forthcoming.

Reflection 13.1. Think about your own health care provider. Do you have an interpersonal relationship with him or her? If so, how do you think your relationship would impact your perception of the provider if you experienced an adverse event? Would you be more inclined to try and understand the provider's views on what happened and why, or would you likely not care, and seek legal action? If you do not have a relationship with a provider, how would that impact your response to an adverse event?

_____

_____

_____

_____

_____

One of the most common causes of legal action that centers on provider–patient communication is a claim of lack of informed consent. Patients who have the mental capacity to make medical decisions have the right to consent to or refuse treatment that is being recommended by their providers.

Incumbent on the provider is the obligation to give the patient sufficient information about the:

- Specific details of the recommended procedure or treatment
- Risks of the proposed treatment
- Benefits of treatment
- Possible alternatives to recommended treatment
- Potential risks of no treatment at all

This information sharing is intended to ensure that the patient can make an educated decision about his or her care. A failure to provide sufficient information needed for the patient to make an informed decision leaves both the patient and the provider vulnerable. Oftentimes, the provider relies heavily on the presence of a signed informed-consent form as proof of informed consent. However, it is critically important for providers to understand that informed consent is not about the form, instead it is about the provider–patient exchange of information (not just from the provider, but via feedback questions from the patient/family). Failure to adequately disclose the risk of certain complications, or fully explain the consequences of a procedure or treatment on the patient's future health can lead patients posttreatment to make a claim for lack of informed consent when there is an unexpected/untoward outcome or adverse event. But effective communication between provider and patient about a procedure or treatment although absolutely mandatory for informed consent must also be accompanied by clear provider–provider communication.

Just as misinformation or ineffective provider–patient communication can lead to legal actions, so too can information exchange errors between members of the health care team. Failures to report or follow up on abnormal lab or diagnostic tests or to communicate changes in the patient's condition have the potential to cause serious harm. Similarly, not addressing provider–provider communication and/or provider–patient interactions regarding a patient's abnormal analytical test or report could result in claims of delayed diagnosis. Furthermore, not escalating a provider's concerns about a change in a patient's signs, symptoms, or condition could lead to claims of failure to monitor and intervene appropriately to protect the patient. Such a scenario could also result in claims against a health care organization for inadequate training and supervision of staff members.

In order to avoid such lawsuits, it is important for providers and health care organizations to have a process or systematic approach to communicating important information to patients. Following up on lab tests that are ordered in the office setting requires providers to train office staff not to file results in the patient record until they have been reviewed and the appropriate provider has signed off on them. Similarly, the reviewing health care professional needs to set aside time to analyze lab and diagnostic tests/reports in a timely manner and then communicate that information to the patient and/ or other providers (e.g., RN, physician assistant [PA], or advanced practice registered nurse [APRN] to physician, or primary care provider to specialist, or vice versa). This expectation includes informing patients of normal tests results (the axiom "no news is good news" should *not* be used in provider–patient communication). In addition, using effective interpersonal health communication to collaborate with patients in their wellness/illness/injury care should strengthen the provider–patient interpersonal relationship. Making it clear that the patient should not be expected to assume a "no news is good news" approach illustrates the provider's commitment to fully informing the patient about his or her findings and encourages the bidirectional flow of health communication and helps to build trust.

Not surprising, it is vitally important for providers to use a systematic process for communicating information with patient-appropriate members of the health care team. Many hospitals have developed systematic hand-off processes/communication policies to ensure that information is not lost when patients are transferred/transitioned between different hospital units/ departments (e.g., emergency department to telemetry, operating room to postanesthesia recovery and/or providers [e.g., hospitalist to hospitalist, RN to RN]). The use of a situation, background, assessment, and recommendation (SBAR), as discussed previously, is one of the communication tools currently used to enhance provider–provider patient-information exchanges. However, many hospitals and other health care organizations have created their own checklist-style communication tools, as well as sign-out/-off formats to achieve safer patient transfers of care and to ensure effective provider–provider (intra- and/or interprofessional) communication. In addition to a standardized format for maximizing provider–provider communication and continuity of patient care, hospitals and other health organizations encourage the use of feedback questions to clarify information that may be confusing or unclear, as well as ensuring assimilation and understanding. Providers need to recognize colleague's handoff questions as being both verbal and nonverbal cues to a potential safety concern and therefore need to ensure that enhanced communication exchanges occur to ensure understanding and resolution of the issue before moving forward in the transition/ transfer of care.

The opportunity for unclear, inaccurate, or omitted provider–patient and/or provider–provider communication to result in patient harm and potential legal liability makes it all the more important for health care professionals to learn and practice effective interpersonal, health, team, and organizational communication, including a focus on enhanced listening skills. The more effective providers' information exchanges are, in all aspects of health care delivery, the more rewarding and less stressful provider–patient relationships will be and the more likely it will be for providers and their organizations to avoid costly litigation. However, it is important for all health professionals to understand the medical malpractice litigation process.

■ ELEMENTS OF A MEDICAL MALPRACTICE ACTION

Lawsuits against physicians and other licensed health care providers based on their negligence when providing medical care and treatment are referred to as *medical malpractice actions*. In order to prevail, an injured patient (plaintiff) must prove the elements of a medical malpractice action by a preponderance of the evidence against the provider (defendant). This merely means that the facts of the patient's diagnosis, treatment, and/or outcomes when presented and given evidentiary weight are more likely than not to favor either the patient's claim or the provider. This is substantially different from the criminal standard, which has a much higher burden and requires proof of a crime beyond a reasonable doubt.

> **Reflection 13.2.** How do you think the differences in the standards for burdens of proof between medical malpractice and criminal acts highlight the need for effective communication even more in health care delivery? Why?
>
> _____
>
> _____
>
> _____
>
> _____
>
> _____

In order to prevail in a medical malpractice action the injured patient must prove the health care provider:

- Owed them a duty
- Breached his or her duty or standard of care
- Breached his or her duty and caused patient harm and as a result the patient suffered damages

Duty of Care

Duty of care is a legal relationship between parties and arises out of the standard of care. A duty of care can be established based on evidence of a provider–patient relationship. Typically, once a health care professional has agreed or been assigned to provide treatment to a patient the provider–patient relationship has been formed. The formation of this relationship triggers the responsibility of the provider to furnish to the patient care and treatment that conforms to the standard of care related to the patient's illness/injury/ situation. The standard of care is defined as those actions that a reasonably prudent provider in the same or similar circumstances would undertake when delivering health care to a patient. All members of the health care team owe the patient a duty of care: doctors, nurses, PAs, APRNs, therapists, pharmacists, and so forth. Their behaviors, not just physicians', must conform to the standard of care for their professions. Similarly, they must act as a reasonably prudent health care professional (RN, PA, MD/DO [doctor of osteopathy], PT [physical therapist], APRN, etc.) in the same or similar circumstances would when providing care to a patient. However, when providers do not follow their professional standard of care for a particular patient's condition, they can be found to be in violation of their professional duty toward that patient.

Reflection 13.3. If a standard of care is that a provider would regularly perform neurological checks (MD/DO, RN, PA, APRN) on a patient who was just diagnosed with a cerebrovascular accident (CVA), do you think it would be a breach of care if no one recorded a neuro-check over a 24-hour period? If so, why? If not, why not? And what does the lack of a reported evaluation communicate nonverbally about the providers for this patient?

_____

_____

_____

_____

_____

Breach of the Standard of Care

As mentioned earlier, when a health care provider fails to offer treatment within the standard of care and it results in harm to the patient, this is referred to as *negligence*. The standard of care can be established in many different ways. When a physician, nurse, or other provider has been sued in his or her professional capacity the standard of care is established through expert testimony. Because most members of a jury lack the specialized health care knowledge and understanding to determine whether a provider should have prescribed a certain medication or used a particular surgical technique in treating a patient, testimony by an intraprofessional peer (MD/DO, RN, PA, etc.) in the same specialty (e.g., emergency medicine, general surgery, ophthalmology) is needed to establish the standard of care in the specific patient's case.

The standard of care can also be established by statutes/laws that define a specific obligation on the part of a health care provider. Hospital policies, for example, can be used to identify the appropriate standard of care when the patient suffers harm as a result of a failure to follow guidelines, procedures, or protocols that were established for safe and effective patient care. It is the issue of harm or injury and how it occurred relative to what is normally done in similar patient/diagnosis/treatment/procedure situations that is critical to the determination of whether or not a breach of duty exists.

Harm or Injury

A patient who has filed a medical malpractice action against a health care provider must prove that he or she suffered harm as a result of the provider's breach of the standard of care. Injuries claimed may include:

- Physical injury
- Emotional harm
- Pain
- Suffering
- Lost wages
- Incurred medical or other expenses for current or ongoing care

In addition, a patient's spouse may be able to claim damages based on a theory of loss of companionship and support (monetary, physical, and/or emotional) because of the injury sustained by his or her spouse. However, it is important to note that the infliction of harm is the critical factor in establishing malpractice. If the patient did not suffer harm, even though there is evidence of negligence, the patient cannot recover damages against the provider. Therefore, in order to prove harm, the patient and his or her lawyer must convince a jury and/or judge that the provider caused the patient's impairment(s).

■ CAUSATION

In order to recover damages a patient must prove that the provider's negligence caused his or her injury or harm. As part of the patient's proof, the injured person needs to demonstrate that the harm suffered was a foreseeable consequence of the provider's actions/breach of duty. The patient *does not* have to prove that the provider knew the harm would occur—only that it was foreseeable to a reasonably prudent provider such that he or she should have anticipated that the harm might occur. When a patient suffers an adverse event, perceives provider negligence, or was injured/harmed in some way, he or she has a legal right to sue the provider(s) and/or the health care organization believed to be responsible.

■ INITIATION OF A LAWSUIT

Few things are as upsetting to anyone as being served with a lawsuit—but especially to health care providers who have spent years studying and committing their careers to helping others. Often the initiation of a medical malpractice action comes as no surprise to the named provider or health care organization. For providers and hospitals, the occurrence of an adverse event, along with the requisite root-cause analysis, to identify what happened and why, also highlights the threat of an impending lawsuit.

However, there are other factors that come into play when a patient decides whether or not to file a malpractice action. As discussed previously, the status and quality of the provider–patient relationship plays a large role in whether or not a patient will choose to file a lawsuit. Based on discussions of interpersonal communication, it should not be surprising to discover that a patient who has an honest, open, and trusting relationship with his or her provider is less likely to sue the health care professional. Conversely, patients who feel that they have been mislead, misinformed, not listened to, or treated in a dismissive manner are more likely to file suit against the provider when an adverse event occurs. Therefore, it is important for providers to recognize that how they communicate and relate interpersonally with their patients will determine in many ways how patients respond when their treatment/condition/procedure turns out not as planned/expected/standardized. The importance of effective interpersonal provider–patient and provider–provider communication in significantly decreasing the risks of a medical malpractice lawsuit cannot be minimized.

Reflections (among the possible responses)

13.1. Think about your own health care provider. Do you have an interpersonal relationship with him or her? If so, how do you think your relationship would impact your perception of the provider if you experienced an adverse event? Would you be more inclined to try and understand the provider's views on what happened and why, or would you likely not care, and seek legal action? If you do not have a relationship with a provider, how would that impact your response to an adverse event?

If you are like many people, how you feel about your health care provider interpersonally will in large part influence whether you may or may not take legal action if an adverse event were to occur. For example, if you think your provider is being honest and open with you, sharing information, collaborating with you rather than directing your treatment decisions—you are likely not to rush to sue. On the other hand, if you see your provider as paternalistic and authoritarian, not listening or seeking feedback, and directing your treatments and decision making with little or not input from you—then why would you not file a lawsuit? Similarly, if you do not have a regular health care provider and have no real continuity of care, it becomes much more difficult to have any concern for someone you do not know let alone trust that he or she is communicating fully and effectively. Therefore, if you suffer harm from someone you do not know well and consequently do not trust—it would be much more normative for you to feel that person has harmed you and should be sued for his or her actions.

13.2. How do you think the differences in the standards for burdens of proof between medical malpractice and criminal acts highlight the need for effective communication even more in health care delivery? Why?

The standards for burden of proof in a criminal case are much more specific and harder to achieve than in a medical malpractice suit. Furthermore, defendants in criminal cases (the accused) can end up in jail; however, in medical malpractice cases—a defendant (provider or health care organization) can have financial consequences—not prison. Consequently, with a lower standard for burden of proof, the needs for effective interpersonal communication and record keeping are even more important for health care professionals. Therefore, to aid in both communication and malpractice risk management, providers need to remind themselves of the importance of documenting their patient conversations, but also their actions, patient information shared with other providers, and what was communicated in order to obtain informed consent. The more effective and interpersonal the information exchanges between providers and patients, as well as between providers and providers related to the patient, the less chance of an error, and the greater the possibility that the patient will not rush to file a malpractice suit if an injury/harm/adverse event occurs.

13.3. If a standard of care is that a provider would regularly perform neurological checks (MD/DO, RN, PA, APRN) on a patient who was just diagnosed with a cerebrovascular accident (CVA), do you think it would be a breach of care if no one recorded a neuro-check over a 24-hour period? If so, why? If not, why not? And what does the lack of a reported evaluation communicate nonverbally about the providers for this patient?

Obviously, the answer to this reflection is in part intrahospital/organization specific. Most health care organizations that care for stroke victims have very specific policies for when patients (based on proximity to the cerebrovascular accident [CVA]) need to have neurologic checks performed and documented by various providers. It would seem unlikely that a patient with an acute CVA, a standard for neuro-checks, would not be evaluated much more frequently than every 24 hours. In fact, depending on whether they are being treated, observed, or prepped for surgery, the neuro-checks could be every 15 minutes, hourly, and so forth. Therefore, it would likely be a breach of standard of care for no neurologic exams in 24 hours, but again, the hospital's/organization's codified policies and procedures would clearly be used to determine what was expected versus what occurred. It is, therefore, important for health care providers not only to know the standards/policies/procedures for care based on the institution/diagnosis/treatment and so forth, but to adhere strictly to them both in terms of performance and documentation (what, where, and when).

Ask someone to take care of a pet for you, determine the SBAR information you need to communicate for your friend/family member to understand the SBAR related to your pet's health, feedings, walks, litter, and so forth. Once you have communicated your SBAR data, how will you be sure that the other person understands? That the information will help keep your pet safe?

Video Discussion Exercise

Analyze the video

- *The Verdict* (1982)

Interactive Simulation Exercise

Pagano, M. (2015). *Communication case studies for health care professionals: An applied approach* (2nd ed.). New York, NY: Springer Publishing Company.

- Chapter 32, "You'll Feel Better Recovering at Home" (pp. 309–318)
- Chapter 45, "I Shouldn't Have to Wait, I Have Insurance" (pp. 423–430)

Health Care Issues in the Media

Hospital adverse event
https://www.youtube.com/watch?v=GEDMYsm3Nxs

Wrong-site surgery happens 40 times a week
http://www.hhnmag.com/articles/4587-wrong-site-surgery

Health Communication Outcomes

Unlike many other professions, health care carries with it enormous risks—for patients and occasionally for providers. As discussed previously, provider–patient communication is often emotionally charged and, based on the patient's illness/injury/quality of life, it can also be confusing and misperceived. However, providers need to recognize not just the health care benefits for the patient from effective interpersonal communication, but also the possible legal value for providers in fully informed consent, collaboration, and shared decision making. Unfortunately, in health care like all other areas in life, unexpected and untoward outcomes occur. For health care providers these situations can result in an adverse event for patients and—if there was provider negligence and harm—patients can choose to sue. Therefore, although it is critically important to deliver the best patient care possible, it is still possible to have unexpected and/or untoward events occur. In order to minimize these, and to provide the best defense possible against a medical malpractice lawsuit, providers need to redouble their efforts to be highly effective, collaborative interpersonal communicators not just with patients, but also with other providers on the patient's health care team. It is important to remember that the timely review and communication of patient's test results and diagnostic reports are just as critical as your examination. Patients have a right to expect to be informed not only of any problems or changes in their diagnostic tests, procedures, or reports, but of the negative/normal findings as well. It is through this patient-centered, participative, and shared communication approach—that encourages dialogue and feedback—that provider–patient relationships can be developed and strengthened with mutual trust to generate an environment that does not encourage malpractice claims when patients have been harmed.

■ BIBLIOGRAPHY

Beckett, C., & Kipnis, G. (2009). Collaborative communication: Integrating SBAR to improve quality/patient safety outcomes. *Journal for Healthcare Quality, 31*(5), 19–28.

Greenberg, C., Regenbogen, S., Studdert, D., Lipsitz, S., Rogers, S., Zinner, M., & Gawande, A. (2007). Patterns of communication breakdowns in injury to surgical patients. *American College of Surgeons, 204*(4), 533–540. doi:10.1016/j.jamcollsurg.2007.01.010

Huntington, B., & Kuhn, N. (2003). Communication gaffes: A root cause of malpractice claims. *Baylor University Medical Center Proceedings, 16,* 157–161.

Institute for Healthcare Communication. (2011). *Impact of communication on healthcare, malpractice risk.* Retrieved from http://healthcarecomm.org/about-us/impact-of-communication-in-healthcare

Lagnese, J., Anderson, C., & Santoro, F. (2015). Connecticut medical malpractice. In *General duty of health care providers* (pp. 1–16). Hartford, CT: Connecticut Law Tribune.

Pagano, M. (2011). Authoring patient records: An interactive guide. In *Legal considerations for authors of patient records* (pp. 89–104). Sudbury, MA: Jones & Bartlett.

Pozgar, G. (2016). Legal aspects: Of health care administration. In *Tort law—Negligence* (12th ed., pp. 63–79). Burlington, MA: Jones & Bartlett.

Rabøl, L., Andersen, L., Østergaard, Bjørn, B., Lija, B., & Mogensen, T. (2011). Descriptions of verbal communication errors between staff. An analysis of 84 root cause analysis-reports from Danish hospitals. *British Medical Journal Quality & Safety, 20,* 268–274.

Skloot, R. (2010). *The immortal life of Henrietta Lacks.* New York, NY: Crown Publishers.

The Joint Commission for Transforming Health Care. (2016). *Hand-off communications.* Retrieved from http://www.centerfortransforminghealthcare.org/projects/detail.aspx?Project=1

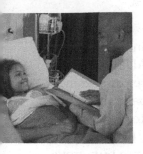

CHAPTER 14

Palliative Care and End-of-Life Communication

For the purpose of this text, we are going to use the following as working definitions:

- *End-of-life communication:* Interpersonal communication (family, friends, providers, and others) that occurs about, during, and after dying

- *Dialectical theory:* The theory that all relationships contain contradictions, some of which are polar opposites, for example, the tension between taking a disease focus versus a patient-centered approach to health care delivery

- *Hospice:* Inpatient or home care for terminally ill patients with the focus on quality of life (QOL) and death rather than disease treatment

- *Narrative theory:* Study of the use of stories to communicate interpersonally about the past, present, and future

- *Palliative care:* Care that focuses on QOL in chronic and/or terminal illness or injury

- *Performance theory:* The idea that humans take on roles, use scripts, and various "faces" to present themselves to others

- *Uncertainty management theory:* A theory that suggests humans balance anxiety and uncertainty in social situations; more specifically, uncertainty about a condition that has serious consequences for more than one person (physical and/or emotional) and the efforts needed to control intra- and/or interpersonal behaviors

■ PALLIATIVE CARE

Palliative care is a branch of U.S. health care that has been receiving more attention in the past 25 years. It actually grew out of the hospice movement, which started in Great Britain in the middle of the last century and moved to the United States in the 1970s, with the first inpatient hospice in Connecticut. However, although hospice care is focused on terminally ill/dying patients with a projected life expectancy of 6 months or less—palliative care extends the focus on QOL in addition to disease/injury treatment for patients (adult/ children) with chronic illnesses/injuries (e.g., kidney, diabetes, cardiovascular diseases, spinal/back/neck injuries, cancers) and for terminally ill individuals. As you might have surmised or witnessed, there are numerous American health care providers who are reluctant to fully support the palliative care goal of QOL over cure. Those providers who are committed to the biomedical model (see *Wit* [2001] for a fictional representation in "Video Discussion Exercise" at the end of this chapter) are frequently unwilling to change their "fix it" lens to a QOL focus. In addition, for many palliative care patients with chronic diseases/injuries, the major impact on their QOL relates to their pain and its management. For many health care providers as well as organizational and government regulators, managing chronic pain is one of the most difficult communication problems they face.

Reflection 14.1. You are a provider working in a clinic or emergency department (ED) and a patient you have not seen before comes in complaining of chronic pain and in need of a refill of a narcotic pain medication. This patient is visiting from across the country and cannot get a refill. How will you use communication to determine the best approach to assessing this patient's request?

_____

_____

_____

_____

_____

Pain management is fraught with numerous dialectical tensions for providers: to treat pain versus feeding an addiction, reduce pain versus create an addict, does this patient really have pain or is he or she just drug seeking? Many providers openly admit that there is a diagnostic conundrum of trying to assess who has pain that requires narcotic pain medication and who is acting. But there is also the potential guilt associated with not properly treating pain versus creating a drug-dependent person (because they have pain that requires addictive narcotics). Nowhere is the communication related to chronic pain and palliative care more difficult than in U.S. emergency departments (EDs). Although the hallmark of palliative care is that patients will have a team dedicated to working with them to address their chronic illnesses and/or pain management—often with written contracts— for numerous reasons these patients end up in EDs and want or need narcotics.

Going back to the previous discussions of the glaring inadequacies of the communication between interinstitution providers and health care organizations in terms of information sharing via electronic medical records (EMRs), this issue is especially problematic for ED providers who want to assess patient's veracity and reported histories. Although it may be possible to check with one or two pharmacies in the area—that is both time-consuming and of little value considering patients can "prescriber shop" and get prescriptions from a breadth of providers and fill them a numerous pharmacies. Although efforts have been discussed to create a true nationally accessible database of narcotic prescriptions for ED providers and palliative care pain managers available 24/7/365, currently there are state databases (for most of the United States), but they differ in quantity and quality of prescription capturing, including how up to date the results are. Furthermore, many states do not share information interstate. Consequently, information that would help providers better assess the needs and realities of patients' pain and pain management is difficult if not impossible to obtain quickly if at all, and this is often in an environment where time management for providers is critical. Unfortunately, drug seekers—and providers know this, which further obfuscates the provider–patient interpersonal communication and increases distrust by both providers and patients. Issues related to health care models and pain management are significant obstacles for palliative care in America.

Based on patients' histories with the health care delivery system, there are often problems in provider–patient relationships that can create additional provider–patient palliative care dilemmas. For example, patients with chronic health problems, by the very nature of their illnesses/injuries, have often seen a number of different providers. Because of their diseases/injuries, the length of their treatments, and their insurance or lack thereof, many of the patients have been passed around among a variety of health care professionals. Therefore, patients in palliative care can be very apprehensive, even hostile because of the way they were treated either by previous providers or the health care delivery system (insurance, hospitals, pharmacies, etc.). Because of these realities, it is incumbent on those providers working in palliative care to avoid stereotypes (e.g., someone who wants pain relief equals a drug seeker) and focus on developing an interpersonal relationship that encourages a patient to share the narrative of his or her illness/injury and treatment. Similarly, providers can analyze patient's communication from a performance theory perspective to assess whether the patient is acting, or using facial efforts to try and confuse or misinform the provider (e.g., appearing in pain, angered by his or her care— past or present—and/or overly emotional). In lieu of an objective record, a national EMR, of a patient's chronic illness, treatment, and palliative care plan, ED and other providers must use their listening, observation, and assimilation of the patient narrative to determine the patient's past and present situation, as well as how best to help the patient until he or she returns to his or her palliative care team or can be transferred to a local palliative care team for evaluation and treatment. It is only through nonstereotypical, interpersonal information sharing that most palliative care patients will receive the QOL assessment and care needed/expected. However, the palliative care of many patients has evolved to what should include hospice care and end-of-life communication.

■ END-OF-LIFE COMMUNICATION

In American culture, few topics are more taboo than death and dying. Children are often kept away from dying grandparents or other family members. The reality that death is a part of the life cycle seems completely lost on most Americans. However, as difficult as it is to talk about death and dying for a large portion of U.S. culture—it is an onerous task for health care providers. Think about it, if you believe in a biomedical model for patient care, then it is indeed accepting failure to treat death and dying as an acceptable outcome for a terminal illness (see *Wit* [2001] in "Video Discussion Exercise" at the end of this chapter for a fictional representation of many providers' responses). In fact, providers' reluctance to accept, let alone discuss, death and dying realities are costing this country millions, if not billions, of dollars (see *60 Minutes* story in "Health Care Issues in the Media" in Chapter 7). However, the difficulties providers, patients, and family members have about openly discussing death and dying issues complicates the need to exchange information—honestly and empathically. Providing patients and family members false hope or insufficient information does little to help the patient make end-of-life decisions regarding estates; postdeath wishes (funeral, wake, cremation, celebration, etc.); and may minimize the time, breadth, and depth of communication they can share with their family and friends. However, providers need to remind themselves that end-of-life communication at its core is interpersonal. Providers need to understand that these conversations, by their very nature, require some additional thought and time for patients to listen, assimilate, and consider. In a culture that shuns death and dying communication and a health care delivery system that sees death as a failure to fix a problem (even though we are all dying from birth), it should not be surprising that providers think there is a death-and-dying script that will help them communicate with terminally ill patients and their families. However, just as there is no one best way to communicate about a pregnancy or a birth (some people are joyful, others shocked, and some distraught), the same is true when having end-of-life conversations. However, there are a few recommendations that may be very helpful for all interactants:

- Try to avoid euphemisms (e.g., *passing away, moving on, terminal, heading to the light*)

- From an intercultural perspective try to avoid religious references (e.g., *heaven, next life*)

- Make sure you have the conversation in a quiet place at a time when you can focus on the patient and not be rushed

- Encourage feedback but make it clear you will come back at a later time to answer questions or discuss further

- Don't offer false hope, especially during/after you have communicated that the patient is terminally ill

- Offer to tell the patient's family (in front of him or her, or in another room) if desired

- If true, assure the patient that you will not stop seeing him or her now that you both know he or she is actively dying

- Be prepared to discuss living wills, advance directives, and hospice care when the patient is ready

Research Question 14a. Find out what a living will and advance directives are and how they are different. What are hospitals'/organizations' requirements regarding honoring these patient documents?

_____

_____

_____

_____

_____

In palliative care and end-of-life communication especially, uncertainty management theory highlights how the unknown and the future become an issue for patients and families. It is important to recognize that patients with chronic illnesses are often uncertain about their health, their futures, and how their lives and families will be impacted. This uncertainty can lead to added stress, anxiety, and depression. Similarly, for terminally ill patients and their families, uncertainty management is often an issue. There are many concerns: from the unknown pain and suffering, to when the patient will die, spiritual questions about an afterlife, and the economic realities of what will happen to spouses and families. Providers can help both patients and their families by allowing them to talk about their uncertainties. Although it is highly unlikely that providers will be able to provide answers to these elusive health care and spiritual queries—for many patients at the end of life, being able to communicate their fears and concerns to someone who is empathic and listens can be extremely helpful. As you recognize the highly emotional and psychologically independent nature of each patient's (and family member's) responses to such a prognosis you will want to be prepared for a variety of diverse reactions. The range of patients' and family members' emotional reactions to a terminal diagnosis, although somewhat predictable, must also be understood and used as a resource for future discussions with the patient and his or her family.

■ ACCEPTANCE IN STAGES

As Kübler-Ross (1969) pointed out, there are often various stages that patients and families go through as they consider a diagnosis and/or prognosis of an incurable disease or injury. Throughout health care and in life, we have become used to getting ill or experiencing trauma and going to a provider or hospital, receiving treatment, and returning to a state of wellness, or at least to an enhanced QOL. However, as part of the life cycle, death is a reality and at some point patients, families, and providers will need to share end-of-life communication to help prepare patients and family members for a patient's death.

Frequently, patients and family members' first responses to a diagnosis of a terminal illness/injury are to deny the possibility. In fact, patients may choose to try to isolate themselves from both providers and family members. The uncertainty, first questioning the prognosis and/or provider's abilities/findings, may be heightened by the patient's fears of pain, being on life-support machines, as well of loss of family and friends, can all contribute to the patient's refusal to accept the diagnosis and to his or her withdrawal from interactions (with providers and/or family). It is important for providers to recognize the patient's need to work through denial, and as Kübler-Ross (1969) and others have suggested, offer to discuss the patient's condition and responses when the patient is ready, but try not to force the patient to confront a terminal diagnosis until the patient wants to discuss it.

Reflection 14.2. Can you recall a time in your life when you were angry about an interpersonal relationship—professional, romantic, or platonic? Did you want to talk to friends about it? If so, what did you want from them in response? If not, how could someone help you through your anger?

_____

_____

_____

_____

_____

When a patient in denial becomes more willing to talk about his or her feelings, a provider may find the patient to be angry. In which case it would not be surprising if the patient is incensed by the fact that he or she is dying instead of others, or that something the patient wanted to finish or do before death is not going to be completed. For providers this can be a difficult time as angry individuals are often hard to communicate with; however, realizing that the anger is not aimed at the provider, but with the disease/injury/circumstances, can make provider–patient interactions easier for both interactants. This stage of death and dying frequently represents a person's view of both his or her uncertainty and realizations that planned/hoped for life events will no longer be possible (sharing time with family and friends, grandchildren's experiences, or even a retirement). Again, the more providers can offer empathic listening, the more patients and families can share their narratives, emotions, and uncertainties—not in an effort to get an answer, but as part of the human condition. However, with time and interpersonal communication, anger can evolve to a dying patient or family trying to use bargaining as a way to emotionally deal with an impending death.

In the bargaining stage of death and dying, it is not uncommon for a patient to want to find a way to make a deal for more time, a different outcome, and so forth. The bargaining phase generally signals a patient's move toward more recognition of his or her condition. It would be hard to make a deal if one did not have a reason to do so. However, the patient's efforts at bargaining may also represent his or her continued attempts to rationalize and accept the diagnosis/prognosis. Providers will need to try to address patient's queries for more treatments, other diagnostic tests, and so forth, with information that helps the patient understand the possibilities if he or she wants to try other options, but also the provider's reasons for recommending or not recommending them. At the same time the provider tries not to offer false hope or treatments, services, and so forth that would increase the patient's suffering, or diminish his or her QOL for however long the patient may have to spend with family and friends. When patients are able to recognize that their diagnoses are accurate and bargaining will not change their prognoses—it is not uncommon for them to become depressed.

Reflection 14.3. Have you ever intrapersonally bargained for something you wanted? Did you ever seek some spiritual help to achieve/attain a desire or goal? For example, some people will internally make a deal like, "If I get this job, I'll stop smoking." Or, "If you save my brother's life, I will go to church every Sunday." If you have used bargaining, how did it help you cope with the emotional stress and/or anger/frustration you had with the situation? If you have not used bargaining, can you understand why a person might use it—especially if he or she has a terminal diagnosis?

_____

_____

_____

_____

It is not uncommon for dying patients and family members to become depressed as they recognize the realities of the diagnosis and the uncertain future looming for everyone. As patients begin to understand that the diagnosis/prognosis is correct and that neither anger nor bargaining will change their outcomes—they frequently become depressed. Again, it is important for providers to recognize the potential for depression in patients and family members. Providers may be able to use their empathic listening as well as their interpersonal communication and relationship building to help patients and/or family members discuss their feelings and uncertainties. Being able to address questions about pain, care plans, hospice, and other clinical and practical issues may be helpful to the depressed patient and/or family. For some, the final stage of death and dying is acceptance.

Providers need to understand that these stages are not a linear plan for patients/families to follow through a death/dying-diagnosis/prognosis. Instead, the individual may begin at one stage, jump to another, not in any order, or go back to a previous stage. Human response to emotional situations is almost never entirely predictable; however, for providers to listen, observe, and assess where a particular patient and/or family member is during a given conversation should provide insights into how the provider can be most effective in trying to help him or her accept the diagnosis and impending death. Acceptance is the final stage in Kübler-Ross's (1969) theory and it is the point at which the patient/family realize and acknowledge that the patient is dying. In this final stage, patients may want to talk more or less, depending on whether they want to share information and experiences or want to be more reflective. Consequently, during the acceptance stage, patients may want to discuss how they will be cared for when the pain increases, or breathing becomes problematic. Similarly, the patient may want to be sure that his or her living will and/or advance directives are understood by providers and will be honored (e.g., not all U.S. hospitals follow patients' do-not-resuscitate directives and instead resuscitate everyone). Also, it may be during this stage when patients want to discuss their funeral/burial/cremation/wake/celebration plans, and/or estate/will instructions. During this time, patients may want to spend as much time as possible interacting with family, friends, but also providers and/or volunteers. During the acceptance phase, many patients just want to talk with others, share their narratives, and learn about future plans for family members, friends, and others. Often, staying interpersonally engaged and involved in discussing either their past or others' futures is one of the ways dying patients communicate their acceptance of their diagnosis/prognosis. Recognizing and helping patients and families communicate in the various stages of death and dying is so important for providers and will be made easier if they focus on a patient-centered approach to end-of-life communication.

■ TAKING A PATIENT-CENTERED APPROACH

Perhaps nowhere in health care delivery is interpersonal communication using a patient-centered approach as important as it is with dying individuals. As highlighted throughout this text, the biomedical model seeks to identify the health care problem(s) caused by a disease and/or injury and fix it. However, this philosophical and pedagogical view of human care puts the emphasis on a mechanistic/investigative view that is highly competitive, depersonalized, technologically driven, and illness/injury-centric.

> **Reflection 14.4.** In order to spend time together instead of watching television, imagine you and your romantic partner have agreed to separately try to solve crossword puzzles every evening. For the first few nights you help each other and talk about your day, tomorrow's plans, and so forth. But then you stop wanting to help or talk, and instead are focused on winning. How do you think that will make the other person feel? What was the goal of this joint effort? Winning or sharing time and an experience together? How might this scenario/approach be somewhat similar to some provider's focus on disease rather than individuals?
>
> _____
>
> _____
>
> _____
>
> _____
>
> _____

Because of the find-it, fix-it mentality of the biomedical model, providers who care for patients using this lens are essentially in a competition—not with other providers but with the etiologic agent (bacteria, virus, failing organ(s), injured anatomy, etc.). Consequently, the provider's focus is not on the individual but on the process that is being sought, analyzed, and/or treated. Therefore, in this competitive, impersonal, health care detective approach, successful outcomes occur when the provider discovers the cause/results of an illness or injury and determines the most appropriate plan for treating it and is successful. However, with this perspective, what are the expected provider behaviors if the illness or injury does not get better or even gets worse?

In American culture we value competitions, and there is generally always a "play/fight/work" to win mentality. Therefore, it should not be surprising in health care that if providers are fix-it focused, they will continue to try to find a solution even when it might be very obvious that the patient will not survive (see *60 Minutes* story in "Health Care Issues in the Media" in Chapter 7). As a consequence, it has been difficult to help providers, especially those who were trained under the biomedical approach, move away from a fix-the-problem-at-any-cost mentality. However, because of the taboo nature of death and dying in this culture, even providers who work under a biopsychosocial approach may not be as patient centered and QOL focused with terminally diagnosed individuals as they are with chronically ill patients. As a result of the delayed or nonexistent end-of-life communication with those patients who have a terminal diagnosis and/or prognosis, those people who might want to make a variety of decisions about the end of their lives are prevented from or delayed in doing so.

There are countless end-of-life decisions that many people would likely want to make if they knew that death was likely imminent. For example, some of the things that Americans have reported wanting if they knew they were dying include:

- Not to suffer, to have the best QOL and quality of death possible
- Being at home with family or friends—not in a hospital
- Discussing with a spouse or family—the dying person's funeral/wake/burial/cremation/celebration preferences
- Putting their financial/estate issues in order
- Sharing time and interpersonally communicating with family, friends, work colleagues, and so forth, but not in a hospital environment

Although it might be possible for some of these things to happen in a hospital, it becomes much more difficult. Hospitals are not designed for dying patients and their families, so rules and environments are not generally conducive to frequent visits, privacy, or patient's freedom (physical and emotional). And although some patients with effective end-of-life communication about their prognosis might initially be concerned that they would suffer without 24/7 nursing care—information sharing about home- or inpatient-hospice care could resolve that. In addition, educating patients and families about living wills and advance directives could be enormously beneficial to helping ensure that patients and families understand the dying person's wishes and discuss how they can best be met. Finally, hospice care in America offers patients and families the possibilities to focus on the patient's QOL and death, while either at home or in a hospice. All too often in 21st-century American health care, because of the lack of open and honest information sharing between providers and patients/families about a patient's condition and prognosis, patients are prevented from making empowered decisions about the final days, weeks, or months of their lives. In fact, although a terminal diagnosis by two separate providers is all that is needed to qualify such patients for hospice care (inpatient or at home), often patients do not receive the information of their expected death until 2 weeks or less before they die and at a point at which they are so weakened and/or ill that they do not get the maximum benefit from hospice, interpersonal communication, or personal reflections. But end-of-life communication is not just about communicating interpersonally and factually with patients—families also need to understand the patient's diagnosis/prognosis.

■ UTILIZING A FAMILY-CENTERED APPROACH

Although Health Insurance Portability and Accountability Act (HIPAA) privacy rules and regulations govern dissemination of patient information end-of-life communication (as well as palliative care) is critically important for families to understand. With a patient's permission, providers should strive to include any interested family members in conversations with the patient about his or her diagnosis, prognosis, and QOL decisions. Generally, it is best not to meet separately with families unless the patient requests it—nonverbally, disparate communication can be perceived by the patient as different information from what he or she was told. Therefore, whenever possible, all patient-related end-of-life communication should be done in the patient's presence. And, although the patient should be the central focus for such interpersonal and group communication, providers need to make such conversations as family-centric as possible.

Reflection 14.5. Can you recall a time when your family needed to discuss something that was difficult—a parent's job loss, a relative's illness or death, or a move? Did that conversation occur one-on-one with a parent and an individual child, or did it take place in a family unit? Which of the two options do you think would be more effective for all and why?

Recognizing the difficulties many Americans have in discussing death and dying topics in general, it is often a bit easier to share information in a group/ family setting. However, providers should consider prefacing their comments by acknowledging the difficulties everyone has in talking about death and dying, especially when about a loved one. Just like patients, uncertainty management theory can be used to assess how families are dealing with the news of their loved one's terminal diagnosis/prognosis. Consequently, providers should take extra time to fully answer questions related to care, pain, QOL issues, hospice options, living wills and advance directives, and so forth. Again, it will be important not to offer false hope or to try to predict the date for a person's death, but instead a provider could encourage family members to talk about their feelings and questions. Also, if the provider will be continuing to see the patient (at home or in an inpatient hospice or hospital setting), then be certain to reassure the family and patient of that commitment. However, the more providers can use empathic listening and encourage family members and patients to share information, the better the opportunity for providers to clarify any misconceptions or miscommunication. Try to help family members and patients recognize the benefits of using the time that remains, not for curative treatments but for QOL/death services, sharing memories, discussing estate and/or postdeath planning, as well as spending as much time as possible visiting with friends and loved ones. Palliative care, especially end-of-life communication, offers health care providers a unique context in which to help patients and families understand that curative treatments are not likely to be successful, but that focusing on QOL (for all) and quality of death (for terminally ill patients) should be everyone's goal. With effective communication, by listening and openly sharing information, providers can use a patient- and family-centered approach to help ensure understanding and a realization of the importance of QOL decisions for patients' chronic and/or terminal health care situations.

Reflections (among the possible responses)

14.1. You are a provider working in a clinic or emergency department (ED) and a patient you have not seen before comes in complaining of chronic pain and in need of a refill of a narcotic pain medication. This patient is visiting from across the country and cannot get a refill. How will you use communication to determine the best approach to assessing this patient's request?

Chronic pain and its treatment create a number of problems for both providers and patients. Because of drug-seeking stereotypes, many providers are reluctant to refill patients' prescriptions—especially if there is no way to check a patient's narrative. For example, late at night or early in the morning when the patient's personal provider is not on call or available, or when a pharmacy is in another state—are factors that complicate accurate prescription data retrieval. ED providers are left to use interpersonal communication to determine whether the patient is receiving or needs palliative care, or is drug seeking. The patient's nonverbal behaviors, pain with movement, exaggerated expressions, and so forth can be assessed by the ED provider. In addition, asking about pain management contracts or palliative care plans may offer some further insight into the patient's history and treatment. However, frequently, providers must rely on their "best guess" and if they believe the patient has chronic pain that requires palliative care, prescribe the appropriate treatment until the patient can contact his or her palliative care specialist. Or if the ED provider is not convinced that the patient is being honest and authentic—then the provider should prescribe whatever treatment he or she feels is needed. Even in 21st-century America, health care is still part art and science and in situations like the scenario in this reflection, providers sometimes need to rely more on the art of assessing a patient's verbal and nonverbal communication and requests because there is very little science to utilize to determine whether the patient is in need of palliative treatment or not.

14.2. Can you recall a time in your life when you were angry about an interpersonal relationship—professional, romantic, or platonic? Did you want to talk to friends about it? If so, what did you want from them in response? If not, how could someone help you through your anger?

For many humans, anger is difficult to deal with because the causative agent or agency may not be clear or cannot be confronted. For example, in a divorce or the dissolution of a long-term relationship, one person may decide to leave and choose not to speak with the other person again. Or when someone commits suicide or dies because of unnecessary risks (e.g., driving while intoxicated), it is not uncommon for those who feel hurt, betrayed, rejected, or abandoned to be angry and not have anyone to communicate those feelings to. When a person is diagnosed with a terminal illness, patients and family members similarly feel angry and uncertain about where to channel/communicate their rage. Providers who understand that anger is one of the stages of death and dying can analyze a dying patient and/or family member's verbal and nonverbal behaviors for signs of the person's fury, but also provide feedback to the individual and offer to listen, discuss, or seek a counselor. The opportunity to express his or her anger and communicate what the patient/family member is feeling can be therapeutic, but is first and foremost a signal to the provider that the patient/family member's fears, frustrations, uncertainties, and rage are not unique and can be helped through sharing their reactions and feelings with providers and others.

14.3. Have you ever intrapersonally bargained for something you wanted? Did you ever seek some spiritual help to achieve/attain a desire or goal? For example, some people will internally make a deal like, "If I get this job, I'll stop smoking." Or, "If you save my brother's life, I will go to church every Sunday." If you have used bargaining, how did it help you cope with the emotional stress and/or anger/frustration you had with the situation? If you have not used bargaining, can you understand why a person might use it—especially if he or she has a terminal diagnosis?

At difficult times in their lives, many humans have made intrapersonal promises/bargains that if they are able to overcome the situation, they will behave differently or act in an opposite way in the future. Similarly, some people try to bargain intrapersonally with a spiritual or religious entity for divine intervention in overcoming a life-changing or life-ending event. For some, bargaining provides a sense of hope that something (e.g., an omnipotent, all powerful agent) will intercede on the person's behalf and change the expected course of events. This perception may indicate that spiritual bargaining is an effort to find hope in a context in which reality dictates that certain outcomes (e.g., illness and/or death) are inevitable. The notion of inevitability with no clear opportunity to intervene, for example, with a terminal diagnosis/prognosis, can lead patients and family members to bargain with providers for "miracle cures" or "trying anything" or with religious or spiritual deities/entities to accomplish what humans are unable to do. If providers understand the role of bargaining in end-of-life communication with patients and families, they can be less dismissive and/or condescending and more empathic and understanding in their conversations. For example, rather than say, "nothing else can be done" or "there are no miracles," providers can try to help patients and families understand that health care has no treatments that can change the patient's diagnosis, but that the future is impossible to definitively predict. Therefore, it might be wise for patients/families to focus on the present, helping provide the best QOL possible for the patient and enjoying their time together. It is to be hoped that by redirecting the patient and family's attention on the present, instead of bargaining about the future, patients and families will not lose the chances they have to fully benefit from whatever time they have together.

14.4. In order to spend time together instead of watching television, imagine you and your romantic partner have agreed to separately try to solve crossword puzzles every evening. For the first few nights you help each other and talk about your day, tomorrow's plans, and so forth. But then you stop wanting to help or talk, and instead are focused on winning. How do you think that will make the other person feel? What was the goal of this joint effort? Winning or sharing time and an experience together? How might this scenario/approach be somewhat similar to some provider's focus on disease rather than individuals?

As you know, masculine-gendered individuals (both male and female), usually have more competitive behaviors. In addition, American culture, with its masculine-gendered focus, encourages competition over collaboration. Therefore, it should not be surprising when the more masculine-gendered partner in a relationship decides to make winning more important than sharing (time, information, or even fun). Although this is often an issue in both platonic and romantic relationships—this "competitive, win at nearly any cost" tactic is especially a problem for providers who see disease, injury, and their complications as problems that must be overcome at any cost (financial, emotional, and/or physical). Consequently, in patients with a terminal diagnosis/prognosis, many providers are unwilling to try and collaborate with patients/families in finding the best QOL outcome versus a continued curative approach. It should then not be too surprising that many more people die in hospitals rather than at home or in a hospice, because providers, especially those using a biomedical approach, want to keep trying to "fix" the problem instead of focusing on what is best for, or might be the decision of, an empowered dying patient.

14.5. Can you recall a time when your family needed to discuss something that was difficult—a parent's job loss, a relative's illness or death, or a move? Did that conversation occur one-on-one with a parent and an individual child, or did it take place in a family unit? Which of the two options do you think would be more effective for all and why?

Many times, family members realize that sharing information, especially about joyful or painful realities, is best done as a group where questions can be asked and answered by all; feelings expressed, shared, and acknowledged; and plans/outcomes/expectations discussed, analyzed and, if needed, collaboratively decided. Therefore, it is often the case that although a parent might tell his or her spouse first about such an event (joyful or sad), rather than sharing individually with children, there is often an effort to bring everyone together to inform, discuss, and respond. Similarly, when it is an adult child with such news (e.g., an engagement, a pregnancy), it is not uncommon for the child to wait for or initiate a family gathering in order to collectively share the happiness or sorrow. Consequently, it should not be surprising for some patients to want to talk about a terminal diagnosis individually with a provider, others to want the news communicated with a spouse/significant other present, and some with their family at their side. As a provider, it would be helpful to find out what the patient prefers, as a terminal diagnosis is a highly emotional communication and, like a cancer or myocardial infarction/heart attack diagnosis, patients and some family members may be so overcome by the connotative meaning of such a report that they cannot process any more information. As with other highly emotional but not terminal diagnoses, providers need to carefully assess their patient's interpersonal communication skills (listening, assimilating, and understanding) based on the conversation's content and the provider–patient relationship. Who should be present at such a discussion is up to the patient (if he or she is mentally competent), but encouraging him or her to consider having a spouse or significant other included in the conversation, and/or other family members as well, may be very important for the patient.

Skills Exercise

Find two people, a parent, grandparent, or older adult, plus a 20- or 30-year-old friend or colleague. Ask them whether they know what a living will is and how it is different from an estate will. If they can provide you with an explanation that you think is appropriate, then ask whether they know what an advance directive is? If they know about both and can describe the purposes, goals, and distinctions between these two health care documents, ask whether they have created one or both for themselves? If yes, why? If no, why not? If one or both of your subjects do not know about living wills and/or advance directives, please use your knowledge to educate the person about these legal documents and why he or she or they might want to consider creating one or both. This conversation is one that every health care provider should be having with all adult patients every time they see them until the patient decides to create a living will and/or advance directive and provide copies to his or her provider to indicate what the patient desires when in the situation/condition described and detailed in the document(s).

Video Discussion Exercise

Analyze the video

- *Wit* (2001)

Interactive Simulation Exercise

Pagano, M. (2015). *Communication case studies for health care professionals: An applied approach* (2nd ed.). New York, NY: Springer Publishing Company.

- Chapter 36, "We Just Need to Get Through the Chemo" (pp. 347–356)
- Chapter 43, "Quality of Life Versus Disease Management" (pp. 407–414)

Health Care Issues in the Media

Opioid prescription database
http://thehill.com/blogs/congress-blog/healthcare/241243-a-national-prescription-drug-database-to-combat-opioid

Dr. Randy Pausch's lecture
https://www.youtube.com/watch?v=-Arnrxle4Gw

The costs of dying in America
https://www.youtube.com/watch?v=F6xPBmkrn0g

Health Communication Outcomes

Palliative care in 21st-century America is focused on helping patients with chronic and/or terminal diagnoses. As opposed to curative treatment, palliative health care is intended to help patients with long-term or end-of-life diseases/injuries have the best QOL/death possible. For those with chronic diseases—respiratory, cardiovascular, arthritis, diabetes, kidney, liver, and so forth and/or cancer, as well as those with debilitating spinal injuries—fixing the problem as is typical in more acute care conditions is not plausible. Consequently, palliative care patients are expected to need care for their chronic conditions for the rest of their lives. Therefore, the hallmark of the palliative care approach is to enhance or at least maintain a patient's QOL. In order to accomplish this goal, palliative care providers need to share information openly and fully with patients, as well as collaborate with them to ensure understanding about the differences in treating a condition/illness/injury for the rest of a patient's life versus curing a health care problem.

One of the main issues that patients and providers have to recognize and communicate about frequently, often including a patient contract, is pain management. Because chronic illnesses and injuries are often accompanied by or result in pain, it is not uncommon for palliative care patients to require narcotic pain management for a significant period of time. This reality is juxtaposed against the continual provider realization that some patients are drug seekers who do not have a chronic illness or injury that requires prolonged narcotic therapy, but rather addicts. This dialectical tension between identifying patients who need narcotic pain medication for palliative care versus those patients who are pretending to have a chronic condition requiring narcotics creates very difficult clinical/ethical/moral dilemmas for providers who are tasked with making treatment decisions with very little prior patient communication/relationship development (e.g., ED providers). However, beyond the chronic therapies and issues with pain management, all of which require increased interpersonal communication, as well as palliative care team communication—perhaps the most difficult in American health care culture is provider–patient and provider–family information sharing at the end of life.

Death-and-dying communication in U.S. culture remains largely a taboo topic. Providers often do not receive formal education in end-of-life communication. Furthermore, the biomedical model that is the focus of many health care providers' approaches to patient care further complicates the provider–patient and provider–family death-and-dying interactions. Consequently, providers often do not want to stop trying to cure a dying patient, even in the face of objective data illustrating the terminal nature of a patient's illness/injury, and therefore delay or avoid communicating the realities to the patient/family. The more providers can accept a palliative care, QOL/death approach to sharing information openly and fully, the easier it will be for dying patients and their families to understand the situation, make appropriate decisions, and spend time addressing the things the patient wants to focus on, rather than ineffective treatments. Palliative care is a long-term approach to helping patients achieve the best QOL possible regardless of the illness/injury/or terminal diagnosis. It is completely reliant on effective provider–patient palliative care team information sharing, support, and collaboration.

■ BIBLIOGRAPHY

Albom, M. (1997). *Tuesdays with Morrie: An old man, a young man, and life's greatest lesson*. New York, NY: Doubleday.

Kübler-Ross, E. (1969). *On death and dying*. New York, NY: Scribner.

Pagano, M. (2016). Learning about dying and living: An applied approach to end-of-life communication. *Health Communication*. (epub ahead of print), 1–10, doi:10.1080/10410236.2015.1034337

Ragan, S., Wittenberg, E., & Hall, H. (2003). The communication of palliative care for the elderly cancer patient. *Health Communication, 15*(2), 219–226.

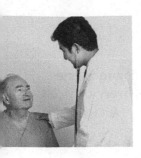

CHAPTER 15

Changing the Culture and Communication of Health Care in America

The purpose of this text is to highlight the critical role communication (interpersonal, intercultural, team, organizational, and leadership) plays in 21st-century American health care delivery. In addition, the current issues related to health care access, economics, quality of care, and so forth are impacted directly by politics, the U.S. health care culture, pedagogy, and a capitalistic approach to illness, injury, and wellness. Just as effective health communication is required for successful patient outcomes, so too is a renewed focus on communication necessary to explore the future of American health care.

■ HEALTH CARE AND U.S. CULTURES

As we discussed in Chapter 5, culture is both created by and transformed through nonverbal and verbal communication. Without shared symbols (language) a culture could not exist. Consequently, American culture is impacted in every way by health communication. Literally, from birth to death, health care and its communication are a part of life for every member of U.S. culture. Not surprising, health care delivery influences not just individuals but every organization and profession, including local, state, and federal governments. Conversely, countless organizations and governments impact health communication and delivery in American culture. Therefore, before exploring ways to change both the macro- (United States) and micro- (health care) cultures, it is important to recognize how the larger culture affects communication and outcomes in health care.

U.S. Values

There are numerous values in American culture; however, a few common ones can be examined to see how they might impact health care delivery or vice versa. For example, Americans value among other things:

- Freedom/independence
- The right to make choices
- Equality
- Privacy
- Free enterprise
- Honesty

As you consider these values, think about the issues we have discussed throughout this book. First, Americans, except for the wealthiest citizens, do not have the freedom to get any kind of health care they want or need. Health care delivery in the 21st century is based in large part on an individual's ability to pay (out-of-pocket and/or insurance) for products and services.

Reflection 15.1. How do you see American values being perceived differently by patients and/or providers in health care than in other consumer areas? Do you feel this is a positive or negative aspect of health care delivery and why?

_____

_____

_____

_____

_____

Similarly, although Americans value the right to make choices, in U.S. health care all too often patients and their families do not have sufficient information and/or shared power to make informed decisions. And, as explained previously, patients do not have equal access to health care delivery based on economic, geographic, and/or communication issues. Furthermore, with health insurers and Medicare/Medicaid unlimited access to their patient's electronic medical records (EMRs), as well as employers' abilities to gather aggregate health data (e.g., anonymous numbers of overweight, diabetic, smokers) on their employees—a patient's privacy is not under his or her to control. Although it would be more normative in American culture for patients/customers to be able to choose which provider, hospital, and so forth they can utilize as in many other aspects of American health culture, patients have only a limited say in their health care options; primarily based on insurer, cost, geography, and so forth. As demonstrated in numerous ways, providers, hospitals, pharmaceutical companies and medical device manufacturers, and others have obfuscated, mis-represented, and/or been duplicitous in their communication with patients, gov-ernment agencies, and/or providers. These differences in modern health care delivery from expected values in America contribute to the communication prob-lems, but also to the dissatisfaction and frustration of many patients, their fami-lies, and providers.

U.S. Cultural Expectations

Americans expect to be able to make purchases and obtain quality products and services for competitive prices with minimal cost, time, and energy expen-ditures. Consequently, U.S. consumers can choose between buying a watch at Wal-Mart or at Tiffany's or having various grades of gasoline to purchase and whether they will pump it themselves or choose a station with an attendant. And for those who want to eat and take as little time as possible, there are fast-food drive-thrus. However, these larger American cultural expectations and realities are often vastly different when customers/patients seek similar opportunities in their health care services. For most U.S. patients and their families, health care costs are difficult to get and obfuscated by point of service (office vs. hospital, outpatient vs. inpatient facilities, insurance copy vs. unin-sured, etc.). Furthermore, although the costs of the same prescription med-ication may be very different from one pharmacy or CVS versus Costco, for example, patients generally do not have easy access to that information and again, it is dependent on the patient's insurer, copay, deductible, and so on. Furthermore, the opportunity for patients/health care consumers to try to choose a provider or hospital based on objective data is extremely problematic, based on the difficulties in matching patient demographics, illnesses, cultural variations, past medical histories, even specific procedures/hospitalizations. For example, there might be a greater incidence of complications (morbidity) and/or mortality in adult pneumonia patients in one hospital versus another. However, that reality may be based on a number of unreported, unknown, or difficult-to-assess factors. It could be that one hospital, based on location alone, gets patients with more chronic illnesses, more immunocompromised patients, or more patients who are homeless and have little or no access to routine care. Therefore, based on location (as most cities require ambulances to take patients to the nearest facility) and patient proximity, one hospital might have a vastly different set of adult pneumonia morbidity/mortality statistics than a similar sized institution across town in a more affluent neighborhood. As you know, health care in America is not equal and this impacts not just access to care, but the patient populations, diseases, complications, and so forth that hospitals and providers are treating. But the difficulties for patients in com-paring and choosing health care providers and hospitals are just part of the reasons why U.S. cultural expectations are problematic for patients, health care professionals, and institutions.

Reflection 15.2. Have you ever asked what it costs for a health care procedure (colonoscopy, appendectomy, etc.) at one hospital or provider's office versus another (not a copay, but the total charge for the service)? If the price for an engine rebuild, oil change, dinner menu, or roof replacement is relatively easy to obtain, why do you think it is so difficult, if not impossible, to get that data from a health care organization?

_____

_____

_____

_____

_____

Because Americans have become accustomed to a fast-food approach to much of life, we expect to be able to get dinner in less than 5 minutes, order a new pair of shoes from our living-room sofa, or get across the country in a few hours, not days. And although it is not uncommon for U.S. citizens to become annoyed or frustrated when their plane is delayed 2 hours, or dinner in a restaurant takes 20 minutes, these attitudes are heightened when it comes to health care expectations. Consequently, not only do patients and their families frequently complain about the length of time it takes to get seen in an emergency department (ED) or urgent care facility, but many are unhappy about the time it takes to get an appointment with a private provider, or how long the wait is in a community health center, or even the time needed to get scheduled for an elective procedure or test. However, one of the most problematic—from a health perspective—fast-food American culture expectation relates to the treatment of illnesses and injuries. Therefore, it is not uncommon for a patient with an upper respiratory infection (also called a "cold"), most frequently caused by a virus, to demand an antibiotic in order to feel better faster (in spite of the health provider's efforts to educate the patient that viruses do not respond to antibiotics and it will likely run its course in the same number of days regardless of the treatment), even at the risk of further increasing the potential for bacterial resistance for everyone. As a result of the differences between U.S. health care delivery and what consumers' are accustomed to in purchasing non–health care products and services, it should not be surprising that confusion, frustration, and anger are often obstacles to effective provider–patient communication. It is clear that in order to improve information exchanges, health care delivery, and patient/customer expectations, health care organizations (private offices, hospitals, pharmacies, insurers, and others) and providers need to recognize these inconsistencies and create mechanisms for improving patients' understanding and access to information, as well as consistent approaches to patient treatment demands (i.e., health focused, not organization/public relations or economically driven). But in the 21st century, patients' expectations based on the larger culture are just one aspect of what needs to be addressed to improve American health care delivery.

Changing the Political Focus

In the United States, health care delivery is closely tied to the government. As noted previously, it was the federal government's intervention in medical education that created the pedagogical opportunities available today. Similarly, federal organizations like the Food and Drug Administration (FDA) and the Occupational Safety and Health Administration (OSHA) strive to protect U.S. citizens from unsafe products and work conditions. And Medicare, Medicaid,

Reflection 15.3. How do you think the disparities in political parties' views, their supporters, and professional lobbyists impact health care regulations, costs, and delivery in America?

_____

_____

_____

_____

_____

and the Affordable Care Act are all examples of congressional attempts to help Americans get broader health care access. But the enormity of U.S. health care costs and the lack of improved health versus other countries that spend far less should be a wake-up call for necessary changes in American policy.

Although the purpose of this text is not to promote one political viewpoint over another, it is important, from a health communication/policy perspective, to recognize that although past and present health care political decisions have created enormous opportunities for providers, health care organizations, manufacturers, and others, patients have not benefited equally. Take, for example, the Reagan administration's decision to close government-sponsored mental health institutions across this country. America's constitution proclaims equality for all; however, we have a health care system that is clearly tiered, unequal, and economically driven. Therefore, health communication is problematic for providers and patients because most discussions have to be based in part on what is financially available for a given patient.

There is no denying that in order to change the culture of health care, we have to change the larger culture in many ways. However, without first having a political vision for what equal health care delivery and access should be in America—it will never be possible. From a negotiation, communication, perspective, what if Congress and the president created a forum to assess the future of health care in America and how it might be envisioned in ways that control costs, but improve access, equality, and delivery? And what if that discussion had one goal, improved quality of life (QOL) and wellness for every U.S. citizen? Then, the specific changes to policies, provider education, nonprovider wellness education, health care organizations, and so forth needed to attain the QOL/wellness goal could be explored. Of course, in a capitalist, free-market country these would be difficult conversations—but isn't the health of the citizens and our national economy going to require them? But one of the key cultural changes such a future would require involves the way we educate health care providers in this country.

Cultural Change in Professional Programs

It will do little good to consider changing the political views and actions of the larger culture, if health care culture is not simultaneously reviewed and altered. For example, as discussed throughout this book, the biomedical/acute/chronic view of health care delivery that predominates in the 21st century is problematic on many levels. By teaching, communicating, and behaving based on a disease-focused approach—providers and patients are for the most part ignoring prevention and QOL issues, in favor of a find-it, fix-it mentality.

Similarly, health care professional education needs to be reconceptualized to better meet the needs of the current health care delivery system, providers, and especially patients. Therefore, if health care in the present and foreseeable future is going to be an interdisciplinary, interprofessional team-focused profession, then we need educational programs that prepare providers to learn, communicate, collaborate, and participate in effective team behaviors. We need to move away from a hierarchical education system that promotes physicians as special/elite members of the team. That is not to say they cannot or should not assume leadership roles when needed, but they also need to be taught the value of sharing leadership, and encouraging and nurturing teammates (intra- and interprofessionally). Perhaps there could be an interdisciplinary health education model, versus medical, nursing, and so forth, with both intraprofessional and interprofessional education. This new paradigm could involve many courses/clinical experiences in which interprofessionals are being trained as a cohort and are learning the advantages of combined education, information sharing, collaborative analysis, and decision making. This team approach to health care education could impact interprofessional acculturation into a wellness/prevention/QOL pedagogical model instead of independent and competing biomedical versus biopsychosocial approaches.

Reflection 15.4. How would you think it would impact interprofessional provider–provider teamwork if health care education was not done in silos (medical vs. nursing vs. physician assistant [PA], etc.)? What would be the benefit of having courses in health professional schools that were interdisciplinary and included an applied opportunity for interprofessional team leadership, collaboration, problem solving, and decision making?

As discussed in earlier chapters, the lack of a prevention/wellness model for U.S. health care creates enormous potential costs, morbidity, and mortality. Furthermore, the disease/biomedical-centric approach of most American medical education leads many physicians focuses on problems that have occurred, instead of collaborating with patients to prevent them and maintain patients' wellness and QOL. Think back to Chapter 12 and the use of risk management in health care organizations. The primary goal of risk management is to identify potential risks and minimize or eliminate them. Clearly it is beneficial to cost, time, provider, and patient/consumers to avoid risks, not to wait until a patient or employee is injured or killed to address the problem. The question is: Why is that different than our approach to health care in general? Would it not make sense and be far more advantageous (for patients and the economy) to work collaboratively, provider and patient, to prevent illness and injury and enhance wellness and QOL, than to focus on treating diseases or traumas after the occur? It would seem logical that prevention and wellness would be the ideal, but beyond the clinical advantages of such a philosophical/cultural shift are the economic realities of the biomedical model.

Reflection 15.5. What do you think would be the differences, from both cost and quality-of-life (QOL) perspectives, in preventing diabetes in later life versus the possible consequences of the disease (e.g., on vision, kidneys, cardiovascular and/or neurological systems)? What impact could enhanced provider–client wellness/prevention/QOL communication in a person's teens, 20s, and 30s potentially have?

_____

_____

_____

_____

_____

Although there have been calls in the past few years to create new payment structures to reward providers who focus on wellness and QOL outcomes versus disease/injury treatments (see Video Discussion Exercise, _Escape Fire: The Fight to Rescue American Health,_ 2013), little has been done to change these practices. The culture of health care and the larger U.S. culture are based on reimbursement for services provided as prescribed in diagnostic (diagnosis-related groups [DRGs]) codes for illness or injury. Clearly, with a health care cultural shift toward valuing wellness and QOL over a posthoc biomedical model—there will still be illness and injury that needs to be assessed and treated. The body is a machine that deteriorates over time, but if the goal is to delay those inevitable changes through wellness and prevention communication and interventions, then Americans could expect not just a longer life, but one focused on wellness and QOL goals. Consequently, in order to overcome the present disease/injury focus a number of key issues need to be addressed, analyzed, and overcome:

1. Physician (and other health care providers) education cannot focus more on diagnosis and treatment of diseases/injuries over wellness, prevention, and QOL.

2. Institution of a compensation system based on provider–patient outcomes is needed; if patients have an equal role in their health care, then they need to be accountable for their behaviors (if economically feasible) and contributions to the agreed upon wellness, prevention, QOL plan. Therefore, wellness would be rewarded at least equally to disease/injury treatment.

3. All Americans need equal access to health care if wellness, prevention, and QOL are going to be universally successful.

4. Continuity of care vis-à-vis interpersonal communication/relationship building by a consistent team of interprofessional health care providers would need to be the norm.

5. Providers would need to be able to communicate with their clients (not necessarily "patients" if wellness is the focus), not just face to face (F2F), but via e-mail, phone, and so forth, without the current legal risks associated with exchanging information without physically seeing a patient.

6. Provider–patient communication and interpersonal relationship-building courses and skills need to be as critical to health care professional pedagogy as biological sciences and clinical skills.

One of the most important shifts that would be required in a wellness, prevention, QOL health care focus is an understanding that effective interpersonal provider–patient communication would be even more critical for success. And therefore, even the language of provider–patient communication would need to evolve. Because the goal would be for providers to work with people who are well—even more than those who are ill, they would not be patients (as currently defined), ergo, a new term would be needed to illustrate the difference between wellness and illness. One term that has been suggested in the past is "client" as in other non health care businesses where professionals work in partnership with clients to meet their present and future expectations/ goals (e.g., tax accounting, marketing, financial advisers). Instead of nearly independent provider assessment, treatment, prescription, and/or administration, a wellness model would necessitate a cultural shift to increased provider–patient communication, education, collaboration, feedback, and follow-up. Thus, the current role of health communication as a tool for providers to gather information (verbally and nonverbally) they need to make diagnosis and treatment decisions (e.g., inspection, auscultation, palpation, percussion, and other diagnostic tests) would need to evolve to at the very least equal provider–client time and effort in sharing information, strategizing, and decision making.

Although it would be an enormous cultural shift to evolve health care pedagogy to a wellness versus illness focus, it could not happen in a vacuum. As discussed previously, political and economic changes would be absolutely necessary. Perhaps equally important, Americans in the larger culture would have to change their views of 21st-century health care delivery and outcomes.

Changing the Culture for Patients

From a patient's perspective, American health care culture has often required a very passive role—parent–child/teacher–student, but almost always subsidiary to providers. This approach has made it easier for providers to control communication and have the power necessary to be directive and authoritarian in their decision making and information sharing. And although providers have been willing if not demanding of this paternalistic style under a biomedical model—it would be nearly impossible for that to be an effective communication strategy in a wellness/prevention/QOL provider–client environment. However, by not demanding a larger role in their health care decision making patients have been complicit as well. They have also been lacking in their self-care. For example, it makes no sense to educate an American about the risks of certain behaviors (e.g., smoking, alcohol or drug abuse, etc.) if they choose (based on their freedoms) to ignore them. This is especially true if the risky behaviors then have the expected/predicted consequences and result in expensive health care treatments (e.g., chemotherapy, surgery, radiation, rehab) that patients are unable to cover (through insurance—private or government, or lack of). These social responsibilities coupled with the economic realities (health care costs to nation, job loss, related family issues, etc.) of their actions, or lack thereof only contribute to our current post-illness/injury/risk problems. In contrast, a health culture that is focused on wellness/prevention/QOL will only succeed if the larger U.S. culture agrees to fully commit to the collaborative work of learning about wellness and prevention, as well as being responsible for adhering to the necessary behaviors to achieve them (e.g., nutrition, exercise, reduced risky activities, etc.).

Just as Americans need a new focus on increased collaborative information sharing and provider–client relationship building, Americans must be willing to individually commit to making wellness the central focus of a new health care delivery system. So too do they need to adapt their illness/injury roles when they do occur. To change the culture of health care when clients become ill, they need to use the information they received as part of their wellness/prevention counseling to help them decide when they need to talk with, or see, a member of their health care team. In order to change the focus from a disease- to a patient-centric health care model, patients need to be much more participative, educated, and empowered. Not every illness requires seeing a provider; however, more communication between patients and provider earlier in the illness may help reduce unnecessary costs, lost work, and frustration (patient and provider). Similarly, it is important for ill individuals to understand the differences in viruses and bacteria and the realities of unnecessary antibiotics, tests, and services. However, this will likely only be possible if providers and clients have time to build relationships and trust during their wellness/prevention/QOL interactions, so that when a client becomes a patient he or she believes the information the provider is sharing and uses feedback questions to communicate his or her concerns.

In addition, with a focus on continuity of care, enhanced interpersonal communication and relationship building, disclosure of adverse events, collaborative decision making, wellness, and more, it is hoped that clients/patients would be more understanding when problems occur. Although there will always be circumstances that require compensation, tort reform is needed so that providers are not paying astronomical malpractice premiums to offset huge judgments. Medical malpractice risks and fears are one of the catalysts for decreased provider–patient interactions—especially outside of the office. As mentioned previously, many providers today will not address their patients health questions on the phone, in e-mail, or after hours, in order to minimize fears of lawsuits. These defensive legal behaviors result in patients being directed to, or going to, the ED for evaluation. Although there are certainly instances in which patients need emergency care, there are also lots of U.S. ED patients who could have been given treatment suggestions over the phone, or recommended to come to the provider's office the next day if they did not get worse. But in view of the litigious nature of our culture and the fact that providers are not compensated for phone calls and so forth, it is the norm for many providers to refer their patients (after office hours) to the ED, rather than discussing the patient's concerns. Patients need to understand that if they want the convenience and rapidity of sharing information with providers via phone or e-mail, they must also understand the limitations for the provider based on proxemics and the lack of an examination.

Consequently, in order to change the culture of health care, including patients' roles and behaviors, effective interpersonal communication and relationships will be more critical than ever before. But politics, pedagogy, professional culture, and patients are still only part of the problems that need to change in health care culture. Organizations also have a major role in the current disease-focused as well as the proposed wellness/prevention/QOL model.

Health Care Organizational Change

In American health care culture, countless organizations contribute to and benefit from the current biomedical approach. Hospitals, long-term care facilities, rehabilitation institutions, pharmaceutical and medical device manufacturers, to name a few all are focused primarily on treating illnesses and/or injuries. Therefore, their communication—provider, patient, and organizational—is disease focused and generally market driven and highly competitive. As difficult as it will be to change health care pedagogy and providers' approaches, as well as patients' roles and behaviors, altering health care organizations' foci on illnesses, injuries, and incomes will be much more difficult.

Although finding ways to change health care in a free-market, capitalistic society is fundamentally monumental, as we have been discussing, the interdependent nature of health culture and the larger culture makes each dependent on the other.

Health care is dependent on the larger culture for patients, products, services, employees, income, subsidies, and so forth. Similarly, health care organizations are reliant on providers, patients, and the government for their income sources. Therefore, if the culture of health care becomes wellness/prevention/QOL driven, it would likely decrease the need for hospital beds, surgeries, ED visits, and so forth. Similarly, with increased wellness, there might be less need for disease-focused pharmaceuticals and medical devices, and with all these decreases comes losses in revenue for organizations, as well as potential layoffs of unnecessary employees; reduced local, state, and federal taxes from the for-profit institutions; and much lower returns on investments for stock and stakeholders.

Reflection 15.6. You are the chief executive officer (CEO) of a large health care system with multiple hospitals or of a major pharmaceutical firm with drugs for hypertension, type 2 diabetes, and gastroesophageal reflux. How are you going to feel about changing the culture of health care to wellness/prevention, both of which will likely greatly decrease your organization's income? Any thoughts about how to use this cultural revolution as an opportunity to enhance your health care organization's opportunities?

_____

_____

_____

_____

_____

Although we are committed as a nation to capitalism, free markets, and independence—the realities of U.S. health care—both economic and clinical outcomes—are eventually at some point likely going to either create a crisis, or a change in philosophy/approach/neutrality. Ergo, it would be enormously beneficial to organizations, governments (local, state, and federal), providers, and patients for leaders from countless health care interests, including patients, to dialogue about how missions and goals of organizations might be retooled, reconceptualized, and/or transformed to focus on a wellness/prevention/QOL future. Instead of making these conversations about winners and losers in such a change, why not seek opportunities to develop a winning outcome for all—especially patients? However, all of these potential changes to U.S. culture and health cultures can only succeed if all members agree to change the focus of health care delivery from a business, income-generating model to a clinical, wellness/prevention/QOL patient-focused approach.

■ BUSINESS VERSUS CLINICAL MODEL

Health communication in America has been obstructed and diminished in many ways, primarily because of the business focus of health care. From providers' fee for service, to insurers, hospitals, technologies, pharmaceutical and device manufacturers, and so many more, American health care delivery is a capitalistic enterprise that is both a huge U.S. budget buster, but also job creator. Although there does not appear to be any ideal template for health care delivery across the world, there are certainly many countries that have far better mortality outcomes than we do for far less expense.

The competition among U.S. health care organizations creates a need to have 25 MRI machines within a 20-mile radius, at millions of dollars in costs, but is that what is really best for cost effective, patient-focused care? Americans are generally willing to drive a few miles to find a service or product they need—why should health care organizations take a one-stop approach for all services regardless of the cost? And remember, the only way a health care organization pays for those technologies is to spread the costs across a variety of products and services. Similarly, pharmaceutical companies, in an effort to minimize losing their research and development costs, almost never do head-to-head comparisons of new products with existing ones in case the new one is not safe or more effective. In addition, the overwhelming majority of new prescription drugs are "me toos," which are safer to create because they are a newer version of a popular product but do not have to be tested against the older version. And with American culture generally preferring the latest product, new "me toos" tend to get prescribed more than the cheaper older versions.

Reflection 15.7. In all likelihood, regardless of your health profession, you finished your degree with student loans. But for the sake of discussion, let's say those loans (college and beyond) totaled $300,000; you now have to decide what area you want to specialize/certify in. If you do primary care, you may earn between 30% and 50% less than if you specialize. How would just those income numbers, and your student debt, potentially impact your post-professional school choice and why?

_____

_____

_____

_____

_____

Another business-related problem for health care delivery and costs relate to provider education. Many physicians finish their medical/osteopathic degree with hundreds of thousands of dollars of debt. Depending on where they did their undergraduate work, it is not unusual for an MD/DO (doctor of osteopathy) to begin his or her residency training with nearly $500,000 of student loans. Consequently, why should anyone be surprised that we have trouble getting MDs/DOs to go into primary care—the lowest compensated specialty in the medical profession? Finally, the business/biomedical aspects of U.S. health care delivery are clearly problematic for effective provider–patient information sharing, collaborative decision making, and improved outcomes. In order to change the current complex problems impacting all aspects of health care delivery—political, economic, clinical, professional, pedagogical, and organizational—a new focus on health communication that strives to create a culture of wellness/prevention/QOL that is patient-centric and outcomes driven is required.

Although there are many obstacles, especially human beings' resistance to change, to refocusing health care culture—there are lots of economic, legal, political, social justice, and, most important, patient/client reasons to negotiate change. Clearly health care professions, providers, schools, associations, manufacturers, organizations, insurers, and so many more will have countless reasons not to attempt this. But we sent Americans to the moon, we eradicated polio therefore, if there is a national will and commitment to improving health care in this country, then everyone will need to benefit from it. And that new health care culture has to begin with effective, honest, communication that provides an opportunity for all U.S. citizens to share their views, analyze options, and find solutions that will make the future health care culture—patient/client-centered, wellness/prevention/QOL-focused, and dedicated first and foremost to improving the lives of *all* Americans.

Reflections (among the possible responses)

15.1. How do you see American values being perceived by patients and/or providers differently in health care than in other consumer areas? Do you feel this is a positive or negative aspect of health care delivery and why?

Clearly, American values like freedom of choice are not possible in today's health care unless a person is so wealthy he or she can afford to pay cash for whatever care by whomever provider. For the remaining 90+% of the country, access to health care is restricted based on insurance, income, and geographic availability of providers and services. Therefore, based on this reality, all Americans are not created equal in terms of health care delivery access to providers and services. These economic and class restrictions and access can be expected to also interfere with provider–patient communication.

Based on the these inequities, it seems rather implausible to expect patients to share personal information with strangers when they are forced by health culture policies to see providers they did not choose (at community clinics, in EDs, hospitalists, etc.), but with whom they are expected to communicate interpersonally and disclose fully their present, past, and family health histories, as well as their social backgrounds.

15.2. Have you ever asked what it costs for a health care procedure (colonoscopy, appendectomy, etc.) at one hospital or provider's office versus another (not a copay, but the total charge for the service)? If the price for an engine rebuild, oil change, dinner menu, or roof replacement is relatively easy to obtain, why do you think it is so difficult, if not impossible, to get that data from a health care organization?

For most Americans, if we want to know what a product, consultation, or service costs, we can ask and get a fixed price or a detailed estimate. Want a 2016 Chevrolet Malibu fully loaded, it will cost $31,915: for a nine-course price-fixed dinner at Per Se Restaurant in New York City, it will be $325 per diner (including service); a meeting with a lawyer about creating a will most likely results in a fixed-cost quote or an approximate estimate, but try to get the price for an ED visit with a strep test, or a prostate radiation treatment—it is nearly impossible because the answers are based on many factors, including whether or not you have insurance or can even pay for the service. These differences in health care delivery are in many ways the opposite of what occurs for clients/customers seeking answers from non health care businesses.

Part of the difficulty in getting concrete prices for products and services in health care is related to our payer system and the disparities in it. For example, the price of a procedure, product, or service will likely be different based on an employer's/employee's health plan, Medicare or Medicaid coverage, self-pay uninsured versus uninsured unable to pay. And, as we have discussed, not only are prices likely different, so too may be the patient's access to care based on his or her plan, financial resources, or a lack of both.

15.3. How do you think the disparities in political parties' views, their supporters, and professional lobbyists impact health care regulations, costs, and delivery in America?

Because U.S. health care policies and regulations are generally politically determined there are often many problems that arise based on the political and philosophical views of the party in power. For example, the Carter Administration passed a 1980 mental health bill that President Reagan overturned when he took office. In addition, pharmaceutical manufacturers, hospital, and provider associations use lobbyists in an effort to influence how members of Congress propose, develop, and/or vote on health care legislation. Therefore, when one party is in power that is supportive of big business theirs is the approach that is generally followed for health care and when the other party, which may be more labor focused, is in power—that will likely influence health legislation. The problem of course is that for citizens, policies and regulations are being influenced and altered based on a variety of interests, which may or may not be the most beneficial to patient's needs, access, and/or wellness/prevention/ QOL outcomes.

15.4. How would you think it would impact interprofessional provider–provider teamwork if health care education was not done in silos (medical vs. nursing vs. physician assistant [PA], etc.)? What would be the benefit of having courses in health professional schools that were interdisciplinary and included an applied opportunity for interprofessional team leadership, collaboration, problem solving, and decision making?

One of the real problems in 21st-century health care delivery is that we teach doctors, nurses, and others providers in completely different programs. Consequently, although this helps acculturate the students into their profession (MD/DO, RN, PA, physical therapist [PT], etc.), it simultaneously supports the distinctions (hierarchical and/or status, education, etc.) among the disciplines (intra- and interprofessionally) and does nothing to help the students once they complete their degrees and immediately are expected to work and communicate interdependently. If new pedagogical models were explored that could both maintain the independent roles with a more applied approach to interdependent, interprofessional provider–provider communication, professionals would have studied and practiced team communication, goals, leadership, and collaboration in a safe, educational context, versus at a patient's bedside/ED/surgical suite, and so on.

In addition, in a more interprofessional education model, some courses could include all providers simultaneously learning how to listen, share information/power/control with each other and with patients as well as learning a common view of the importance of a patient-centered focus on wellness/prevention/QOL. If providers are going to be working more and more in teams in hospitals and wellness clinics, helping them prepare for the various team roles (leader, follower, problem solver, idea generator, etc.) they will need to use in various situations can only decrease the stress of current health care delivery and enhance the trust, relationship building, and communication climate needed for effective and supportive health care teams.

15.5. What do you think would be the differences, from both cost and quality-of-life (QOL) perspectives, in preventing diabetes in later life versus the possible consequences of the disease (e.g., on vision, kidneys, cardiovascular and/or neurological systems)? What impact could enhanced provider-client wellness/prevention/QOL communication in a person's teens, 20s, and 30s potentially have?

This is a philosophical conundrum and illustrates the dialectical tensions between what Americans want in terms of freedom of choice and what happens when citizens' choices result in negative consequences for their health, as well as the economic costs of their behaviors for U.S. culture. For example, to offset some of the costs to society from smoking, cigarettes are highly taxed. And while it can be argued that the money collected from smokers can help pay for some of the pulmonary and cardiovascular consequences of long-term tobacco use if the patient is on Medicare or Medicaid. However, many smokers are likely not eligible for Medicare or Medicaid and instead are enrolled in an employer health insurance plan that is paying for their care until age 65, or whenever they retire or are too sick to work. Therefore, this tobacco tax money is not supporting the employee members of the smokers' insurance plan who are being charged higher premiums and copays based on the number of enrolled who have chronic illnesses, and/or exacerbations of chronic pulmonary problems by continued smoking (ED visits, medications, treatments, diagnostic tests, etc.). Consequently, while Americans have the right and freedom to behave legally any way they choose, there are very significant consequences to known risky health behaviors and as we strive to reduce health costs and improve wellness and QOL it is important to realize that not only the smoker's QOL is being impacted by their decisions, but hypothetically, hundreds, thousands, even tens of thousands and eventually millions of Americans who are part of the same health plan and/or taxpayers when smokers have to rely on government plans for coverage. The health of U.S. citizens creates real dialectical tensions: philosophically, economically, and politically for all Americans.

15.6. You are the chief executive officer (CEO) of a large health care system with multiple hospitals or of a major pharmaceutical firm with drugs for hypertension, type 2 diabetes, and gastroesophageal reflux. How are you going to feel about changing the culture of health care to wellness/prevention, both of which will likely greatly decrease your organization's income? Any thoughts about how to use this cultural revolution as an opportunity to enhance your health care organization's opportunities?

For health care organizations of all types, change is both necessary and problematic. If you are the CEO of a large health care system, you are likely concerned about how your disease-focused, acute care model can survive in a wellness/prevention/QOL culture. However, not only will there always be patients who need acute and chronic care, a strategic CEO might see such a change as a way to reinvent how his or her organization provides care. Consequently, it might be that the more futuristic institutions develop health outcome rubrics that reward providers and organizations their wellness/prevention/QOL effectiveness—as much or more as their disease treatment. Clearly, it will be easier for a CEO or an organization to find all the problems and risks in changing its mission, values, and goals, but at the same time, hospitals and health care organizations have been evolving constantly over the past 100-plus years. The key is to identify what their consumers/clients/patients want and/or need and find the best way to meet those needs/expectations in order to grow in a changing health care culture.

15.7. In all likelihood, regardless of your health profession, you finished your degree with student loans. But for the sake of discussion, let's say those loans (college and beyond) totaled $300,000; you now have to decide what area you want to specialize/ certify in. If you do primary care, you may earn between 30% and 50% less than if you specialize. How would just those income numbers, and your student debt, potentially impact your post-professional school choice and why?

If you are like most Americans, earning a higher income is likely one of your goals. In addition, if you have to repay $300,000 in student loans, would it not make more sense to choose the highest paying career? And, in the current health care culture, if you specialize you likely will be perceived as having a higher status than those who are in primary care. Consequently, our current health care delivery environment and culture promotes specialization from both status and income perspectives. The question for the future is how does the health care culture change the focus for providers to one that compensates primary care providers, as well as other certified/specialists, in ways that make it not only economically beneficial to be a primary care provider, but desirable as well?

Skills Exercise

Ask some of your health care provider friends, colleagues, or professors what they see as the future for patient care in America. Do they think it needs to change? If so, why and how? If not, why not? Based on this chapter, pick a topic to discuss with them as possible changes and see what feedback you get and how you respond.

Video Discussion Exercise

Analyze the video

- *Rx: The Quiet Revolution* (2015)
- *Escape Fire: The Fight to Rescue American Health* (2013)

Interactive Simulation Exercise

Pagano, M. (2015). *Communication case studies for health care professionals: An applied approach* (2nd ed.). New York, NY: Springer Publishing Company.

- Chapter 28, "We Need to Improve Our Press Ganey Scores" (pp. 275–282)
- Chapter 43, "Quality of Life Versus Disease Management" (pp. 407–414)

Health Care Issues in the Media

The three trillion dollar health care system
http://www.nytimes.com/2015/12/03/us/politics/health-spending-in-us-topped-3-trillion-last-year.html?emc=eta1

Health Communication Outcomes

This book has focused on a variety of provider–patient, provider–provider, and provider–organization health communication behaviors in diverse cultures and contexts (dyadic, team, office, hospital, larger culture). In addition, the impact of politics, culture, economics, pedagogy, and capitalism on effective health communication sharing and outcomes has also been explored. However, as illustrated in this text, the past and present predominant use of a disease-focused, provider-centric, biomedical model serves only to minimize the potential for and/or discourage patient collaboration. Furthermore, perhaps even patients' commitment to health/wellness behaviors are being negatively impacted by what they perceive as paternalistic determination and communicaion, with few options for other perspectives/access. Consequently, based on these observations and realities, changing the future of health care delivery requires altering the culture and communication of 21st-century American wellness, illness, and injury.

The culture of health care in America is vastly different from other aspects of people's lives. For example, the costs and access to health care are far more obfuscated and tiered versus other non–health care products, services, and organizations. In addition, traditional American values of freedom of choice and equality are not part of the U.S. health care delivery system. Patients' choices are driven economically in large part; we have a financially tiered system of health care access—based on a person's ability to self-pay, type of health insurance, or the lack of insurance and/or income. In addition, political decisions, regulations, and laws all influence health care delivery but appear to be based more on the political party in control, corporations'/lobbyists' stimuli, and/or economic realities, versus consumers'/citizens'/patients' needs and/or expectations. However, in addition to the culture and politics that markedly impact health communication and patient care—there is also the role that professionals, pedagogy and U.S. patients play in information exchanges, shared decision making, and enhanced QOL outcomes.

The focus on providers and the biomedical model is often the central aspect of many health profession education programs (MD/DO especially). Consequently, to change the health care culture in America, a new patient-centric wellness/prevention/QOL focus will be necessary. However, it will not be enough to just change the philosophical and educational foci of health professional pedagogies, there needs to be a reconceptualization of how hierarchy and status are communicated and viewed in order to help providers both intra- and interprofessionally in team and provider–provider communication. Similarly, changing providers' foci and approaches without concurrent efforts to alter patients' health care behaviors will likely be unsuccessful. Too often patients choose not to trust, understand, or follow providers' and other health care educational messages (e.g., smoking, obesity, addiction risks). And, although it could be argued that this results from the current inequities in health care access and communication, it also can be in part attributed to individuals who are purposefully choosing to behave (e.g., American freedom) in ways that are not only unhealthy (e.g., nutrition, exercise, medications—prescribed and not taken or inappropriate/addictive) but self-destructive. These behaviors frequently lead to increasing U.S. health care costs to cover the acute and chronic health care expenses resulting from such decisions/behaviors. However, it needs to be stated that these chosen unhealthy behaviors are distinct from nutrition, shelter, and other health-related behaviors that some Americans are forced to endure based on limited access to care and/or finances that prevent more nutritious meals, lodging, and life choices. If America is to change the focus of health care to a wellness/prevention/QOL model, it needs to be supported and enacted by the health care culture and entire larger culture, including health care professionals' education, providers, patients, and politicians. However, major health care cost drivers—service providers, product manufacturers, and other health care organizations—will also need to be willing to explore diverse approaches to changing health care delivery and communication.

Health care organizations, hospitals, nursing homes, rehabilitation centers, providers offices, product manufacturers, and countless others have markedly profited from the current biomedical, disease-focused approach to patient care. Therefore, it will not only require considerable mission and goal revisions for these institutions, it will require potential financial losses if they cannot find ways to contribute to a new wellness/prevention/QOL, patient-centric focus. Consequently, in order to effect these transformational changes, U.S. citizens will have to be not only supportive, but also demonstrative through their election decisions and their health care purchases/choices. In order to have any chance in the relatively near future of changing U.S. health care delivery from a disease-focused, business-driven model to a patient-centered, wellness/prevention/QOL approach, numerous aspects of American culture must change. In order to move to a health care delivery system that values effective information sharing, equal access, collaborative decision making, and compensation based on health outcomes, not services/products provided, America will need to openly discuss the necessary cultural, political, economic, business, and societal changes that would need to be enacted. It will take extensive and effective interpersonal, political, interorganizational, and inter-professional discussions/negotiations if we want to improve U.S. health care delivery, health communication, wellness, and QOL outcomes—but it cannot happen if Americans don't begin the conversation.

■ BIBLIOGRAPHY

Cassells, A. (2012). *Seeking sickness: Medical screening and the misguided hunt for disease.* Vancouver, BC: Greystone Books.

Gawande, A. (2007). What doctor's owe. In *Better: A surgeon's notes on performance, Part II.* New York, NY: Picador.

Horstmann, S. (2013, September 13). When nurses bond with their patients. *New York Times.* Retrieved from http://nyti.ms/18WK6Js

Korsch, B., & Negrete, V. (1972). Doctor patient communication. *Scientific American, 27,* 66–74.

Pagano, M. (2011). *Authoring patient records: An interactive guide.* Sudbury, MA: Jones & Bartlett.

Peckham, C. (2015). *Medscape physician compensation report 2015*. Retrieved from http://www.medscape.com/features/slideshow/compensation/2015/public/overview#page=3

Thomas, A. (1998). Ronald Reagan and the commitment of the mentally ill: Capital, interest groups, and the eclipse of social policy. *Electronic Journal of Sociology*, 3(4). Retrieved from http://sociology.org/content/vol003.004/thomas_d.html

Welch, H. (2015). *Less medicine more health: 7 assumptions that drive too much medical care*. Boston, MA: Beacon Press.

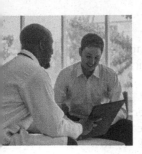

Index

Printed in the United States
By Bookmasters